Designer: Katie Kelly
Medical proofreader: Aneida Skeens
Printer: Createspace

Copyright © 2014 Wallace Digital Media
PO Box 425
Newtown, Pennsylvania 18940

All rights reserved. This book is protected by copyright. No part of this book may be reproduced in any form or by any means, including photocopying without written permission form the copyright holder.

The publisher and author are not responsible (as a matter of product liability, negligence, or otherwise) for any injury resulting from any material contained herein. This publication contains information relative to general principles of medical care and should not be construed as specific instruction for individual patients. Manufacturer's product information and package inserts should be reviewed for current information, including contraindications, dosages and precautions.

The publisher and author are not responsible (as a matter of product liability, negligence, or otherwise) for individual exam results. This publication should not be considered a comprehensive review for the PANCE or the PANRE and should be used in conjunction with additional resources.

The publisher has made every effort to avoid any copyright infringement through out this publication. If there is anything that may have been inadvertently overlooked please contact **support@physicianassistantexamreview.com** and we will be happy to resolve the situation as soon as possible.

If you have any question as to the accuracy of any information in this book please contact **support@physicianassistantexamreview.com** and we will attempt to resolve the matter as quickly as possible.

Thank You!

I want to take a moment right at the beginning to say THANK YOU! Your purchase of the *The Final Step* makes a huge impact, not only on you and me, but on the entire PA community.

By purchasing the *The Final Step*:

- ✓ <u>You</u> get a valuable tool to use in preparing for your test. I believe there is no better resource you can use in in the week leading up to your exam.

- ✓ <u>You</u> help me take Physician Assistant Exam Review from a hobby, which took time and energy away from my family, and change it into a resource that helps support them.

- ✓ <u>You</u> allow me to continue to create great FREE content on **www.physicianassistantexamreview.com**, including the podcast and study notes, for the entire PA community.

For all of this, thank you. If you know of anyone else who would like to boost their confidence for exam day please send them to www.physicianassistantexamreview.com/thefinalstep to pick up their very own copy.

Sincerely,

Brian, Betty, Colin and Derek Wallace

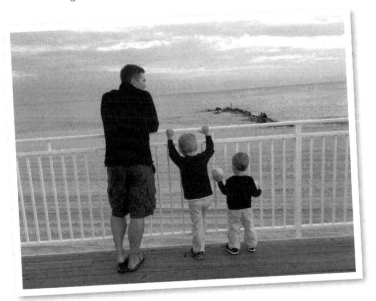

To my wife, Betty, you believed in me even when I didn't believe in myself. This and so so many other things would not be possible without you.

To the PAER community, your help getting this project off the ground can not be overstated. Your requests for this resource, your continued help with editing and the encouragement of your successes have kept me going. I'm sure I would leave someone out if I named names, so I'm just going to say **thank you**.

Brian Wallace

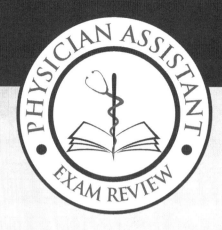

This book was initially written while I was studying for my PANRE. It is designed specifically as an aid for passing your exam and not for clinical practice. The questions cover the most important information you need to know as quickly as possible. I used these key questions to review at the end of each topic and then again to review everything just before my exam. That's where the title *The Final Step* comes from.

You will find that the questions are very short. The idea is to be able to review as many key ideas as possible in as short a time period as possible. These questions are designed to be used only after you feel comfortable with the content of each topic. You should use several different resources while preparing for your exam, and the *The Final Step* will take you across the finish line.

The Final Step is split into two sections. The first has the questions divided by topic. This is designed so that you can easily quiz yourself at the end of a study session. Section B is all 1200 questions in a completely random order. This section is best used in the days leading up to your exam when you want to cover everything as fast as possible.

This book has helped hundreds of students and PA's pass their exams, and I am confident it will do the same for you. Thank you and good luck!

      Brian Wallace, PA-C

TABLE OF CONTENTS

Section A

Musculoskeletal 6
Neurology 13
Psychology 20
Cardiology 26
Dermatology 41
Endocrinology 45
ENT 51
Genitourinary 55
Hematology 60
Infectious Disease 63
Ob-Gyn 71
Ophthalmology 82
Pulmonology 87
Gastrointestinal 94
Pediatrics 103

Section B

All 1200 questions and 15 topics
in random order 108

MUSCULOSKELETAL

- At what age should you begin ordering dexa scans for male patients? What about female patients?

    70 for males, 65 for females

- Give the DEXA score for osteopenia and Osteoporosis.

    Osteopenia = 1 to 2.4 standard deviations, osteoporosis = 2.5 standard deviations or greater

- What fracture is the #1 cause of compartment syndrome?

    Tibial shaft fracture

- A patient's lab work shows positive Smith antibody and positive double-stranded DNA antibodies. What is the most likely diagnosis?

    Lupus

- Where are Bouchard's nodes found?

    Proximal interphalangeal joint (PIP)

- What will an x-ray show in acute osteomyelitis?

    Nothing - it will show bone destruction in chronic osteomyelitis.

- What is the best imaging to diagnose osteomyelitis?

    Either a bone scan or an MRI will provide the diagnosis.

- A 22 year old male patient presents with what is clearly a septic knee. You also notice lesions on his hands and feet. What is the most likely pathogen?

    Neisseria gonorrhoeae

- What would you expect the WBC count to be in the joint fluid of an infected knee?

    >50,000 at a minimum and probably much higher.

- A patient presents with a painless mass in her right wrist. What is the most likely diagnosis?

    Ganglion cyst

- What is the age range for osteosarcoma? Where are they most typically found in the body?

    Osteosarcoma usually occur in 15-25 year old males and are most commonly found around the knee.

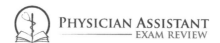

MUSCULOSKELETAL

- You think a patient may have an osteoid osteoma due to his complaints of severe night pain. You set him up for an x-ray; but in the meantime what medication do you start him on?

    If it is truly an osteoid osteoma ibuprofen will resolve his pain.

- Clicking or locking of the knee indicates what diagnosis?

    Meniscal tear

- A 65 year old presents complaining of severe pain in his great toe that began when he woke up this morning. It is swollen, red and very tender. What is the most likely diagnosis?

    Gout would be number one because of the location, but you might also think about an infection.

- What uric acid level helps to confirm a diagnosis of gout?

    >7.5

- What is the medical treatment for gout?

    Allopurinol, colchicine

- A pathology report comes back with positive birefringent crystals. What is the most likely diagnosis?

    Pseudogout

- A patient with a history of hepatitis B presents complaning of bilateral knee pain, fever and weight loss. What is the most likely diagnosis?

    Polyarteritis nodosa

- You suspect a patient has polyarteritis nodosa. What is the test for a definitive diagnosis and what is the treatment?

    Biopsy, high dose steroids

- On physical exam, you notice ulnar deviations and swan neck deformities. What is the most likely diagnosis?

    Rheumatoid arthritis

- A positive Neer's test indicates what diagnosis?

    Rotator cuff impingement

- List three medication that may cause lupus.

    Procainamide, isoniazid and Quinidine

MUSCULOSKELETAL

- What test do you do for Sjogren's syndrome?

  Schirmer test

- A patient with rheumatoid arthritis is heading to the OR for open reduction and internal fixation of the ankle. In addition to ankle films, what other x-rays should you get?

  C-spine, anesthesia will want them due to concerns about instability of C1 & C2.

- Which carpal bone has a high rate of nonunion and occult fracture?

  Scaphoid

- What medication is used for patients with lupus?

  Systemic steroids

- Scleroderma limited version has five main characteristics for which the CREST acronym is often used. What are those five things?

  Calcinosis, Raynaud's, esophageal dysmotility, Sclerodactyly, Telangiectasia

- There is a sunburst appearance on x-ray. What is the most likely diagnosis?

  Osteosarcoma

- Anatomically where are 80% of clavicle fractures located?

  Middle third

- A pathology report comes back showing negatively birefringent crystals. What is the most likely diagnosis?

  Gout

- What are the four muscles of the rotator cuff?

  Commonly referred to as the SITS muscles they are Supraspinatus, Infraspinatus, Teres minor, Subscapularis.

- Describe the characteristics of a lytic lesion on x-ray.

  Spiculated, elevated periosteum, bone destruction (think bad, very bad things)

- What ligament is most commonly injured in an ankle sprain?

  Anterior talofibular ligament (ATFL)

MUSCULOSKELETAL

Vasculitis with a hepatitis B history should make you think of what diagnosis?	Polyarteritis nodosa
What is the most common fracture in children?	Clavicle
A fat pad sign on a lateral x-ray of the elbow has what significance?	It is blood in the joint indicating a fracture even if the fracture line cannot be seen.
A patient presents with progressive neck and proximal muscle weakness. On physical exam, you see a reddish purple maculopapular rash. Her lab work shows an anti-Jo-1 antibodies. What is the most likely diagnosis?	Polymyositis
Which way does a Colles fracture angulate: dorsal or volar? What about a Smith fracture?	Colles = Dorsal, Smith = Volar
Tenderness over the anatomical snuffbox is indicative of what fracture?	Scaphoid
What is the most common fracture in a patient with osteoporosis?	A compression fracture of a vertebral body followed by hip fractures.
A 15 year old boy presents complaining of night pain in the pelvis. Since you have no idea what to do, you order an x-ray. The report comes back with a description of a mass with an "onion skin appearance." What is the most likely diagnosis?	Ewing sarcoma
What is the name for the 4th and 5th metacarpal fractures that often result from throwing a punch?	Boxer's fracture
A new mother presents with pain over the radial wrist. She has a positive Finkelstein's test. What is the most likely diagnosis?	de Quervain's tenosynovitis
A positive McMurry indicates what diagnosis?	Meniscal tear

MUSCULOSKELETAL

What is the first line treatment for carpal tunnel?	Night splint
What is the most common cause of C-spine fractures?	Motor vehicle accidents
What is the medical term for hunchback?	Kyphosis
What is another term for podagra?	Gout
A patient presents to the ER with saddle anesthesia and loss of bowel and bladder function. What is the most likely diagnosis?	Cauda equina
A patient with HIV presents with severe groin pain. What is the most likely diagnosis?	Avascular necrosis of the femoral head. Antiretroviral medications put patients at an increased risk of AVN.
A 95 year old female presents to ER after a fall in her home. Her left leg is shortened and externally rotated. What is the most likely diagnosis?	Hip fracture
You recommend bisphosphonates for a patient with osteoporosis. What instruction do you give her for immediately after taking the medication?	Remain upright for 30 minutes
What is the most common cause of a hip dislocation? Is it usually anterior or posterior?	MVA, posterior
Which of the four rotator cuff muscles is most commonly injured?	Supraspinatus
What is the medical term for tennis elbow?	Lateral epicondylitis
What is a first line treatment for rheumatoid arthritis?	Methotrexate
A patient presents to the ER after taking a baseball bat to the knee. He is unable to actively extend his knee. What is the most likely diagnosis?	Patella fracture

MUSCULOSKELETAL

Are most shoulder dislocations anterior or posterior?	*Anterior*
What is the most useful physical exam test for diagnosing an ACL tear?	*Lachman's, followed by anterior drawer*
What is the most common knee injury?	*Medial meniscal tear*
Where are Heberden's nodes found?	*Distal interphalangeal joint (DIP)*
A patient presents with knee pain following a soccer game two days ago. He has joint line tenderness medially and feels a locking in the knee from time to time. What two physical exam tests should you do?	*This is probably a medial meniscal tear. McMurry and apply tests would be appropriate.*
A patient presents with conjunctivitis, urethritis, arthritis and oral lesions. What is the most likely diagnosis? What other lab might you expect to be positive?	*Reactive arthritis, HLA B-27*
A 46 year old male comes into ER limping a little on the right side. He states that it felt as though he was kicked in the back of the leg during a soccer game, but clearly no one was behind him. What is the most likely diagnosis?	*Achilles tendon rupture*
Anti-Jo-1 antibodies should make you think of what diagnosis?	*Polymyositis*
A positive crossover test indicates what diagnosis?	*Acromioclavicular joint injury (AC joint)*
A positive Hawkins test indicates what diagnosis?	*Rotator cuff impingement*
A positive Finkelstein's test indicates what diagnosis?	*de Quervain's tenosynovitis*

MUSCULOSKELETAL

- A positive Phalen and Tinel's sign indicates what diagnosis?

    Carpal tunnel

- A bamboo spine indicates what diagnosis?

    Ankylosing spondylitis

- A positive straight leg test indicates what diagnosis?

    Herniated disc

- An African American female presents with malar rash and a positive double-stranded DNA antibody. What is the most likely diagnosis?

    Lupus

- Carpal tunnel affects what nerve and what parts of the hand?

    Median nerve. Thumb, pointer and ring fingers. Thenar wasting is sign of advanced disease.

- A patient has a silver-fork deformity on x-ray. What is the most likely diagnosis?

    Colles fracture

- A positive Apley indicates what diagnosis?

    Meniscal tear

NEUROLOGY

- List six medications that can be used for migraine prophylaxis?

    Beta blockers, tricyclics, calcium channel blockers, NSAIDs and valproic acid

- A patient presents with what appears to be an inability to understand speech. Which aphasia should be at the top of your differential?

    Wernicke's aphasia

- A patient presents with facial paresis, arm drift and abnormal speech. What are the first three tests to order?

    Thinking of a stroke you order a non-contrast brain CT or MRI, serum glucose and oxygen saturation.

- A patient is brought in following a seizure in which she did not lose consciousness. What is the most likely diagnosis?

    Simple partial seizure

- A patient is having a stroke and there is no evidence of hemorrhage. What is the first line medical treatment?

    Within the first 4 hours and with no contraindications thrombolytics should be given.

- A patient presents with a painful ipsilateral third nerve palsy. What is the most likely diagnosis?

    Posterior communicating artery aneurysm (PComA)

- What siezure medication may cause overgrowth of the gums?

    Phenytoin

- A sudden thunderclap headache should make you think of what diagnosis?

    Subarachnoid hematoma

- Describe Kernig's sign.

    The patient lies supine, flex hip while keeping knee straight. Back pain is positive.

- Imaging is negative for blood, but you strongly believe that there is a subarachnoid hemorrhage. What test can you order that will be definitive?

    Lumbar puncture

NEUROLOGY

- [ ] A patient presents with a lateralized throbbing headache. He is also complaining of nausea, vomiting and photophobia. What type of headache is most likely?

    Migraine

- [ ] A middle age male presents with unilateral periorbital headaches occurring daily for several weeks. These headaches are extremely painful. Which type of headache is the most likely cause?

    Cluster headache

- [ ] List three drugs that treat cluster headaches.

    Oxygen, sumatriptan, Stadol (butorphanol)

- [ ] A 34 year old presents with symptoms which are relapsing and remitting over the past few weeks. These include visual problems and weakness in her right arm. What is the most likely diagnosis?

    Multiple sclerosis

- [ ] A patient has a tremor with motion in his hands. What medication might you prescribe?

    This patient has an active tremor. A beta blocker like propranolol is a good start.

- [ ] A shuffling gait should make you think of what diagnosis?

    Parkinson's disease

- [ ] Give two classes of drug therapy for treating Parkinson's.

    Dopaminergic (levodopa), anticholinergics are second line

- [ ] Decreased GABA and substance P should make you think of what diagnosis?

    Huntington's

- [ ] Is Huntington's autosomal dominant or recessive?

    Dominant

- [ ] A patient presents with weakness that he has felt in his lower legs and now feels in his knees and hips bilaterally. He has decreased deep tendon reflexes. This has been getting progressively worse. What is the most likely diagnosis?

    Guillain-Barre

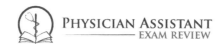

NEUROLOGY

- What percentage of strokes are ischemic? What percentage are hemorrhagic?

    80%, 20%

- You believe a patient has had a stroke. He presents with aphasia, loss of hearing in one ear and loss of vision in his left eye. Is the blockage likely in the anterior or posterior circulation?

    Anterior

- Under what conditions would aspirin or clopidogrel be used following a TIA as prophylaxis?

    These are antiplatelet medications. They would be used unless there is a known cardiac etiology for the embolism. Patients with a cardiac cause should use heparin or Coumadin.

- A patient who is asymptomatic should consider having an endarterectomy at what percent blockage of the carotid artery? How about in a symptomatic patient?

    70% in an asymptomatic patient and greater than 60% in a symptomatic patient.

- A patient presents complaining of the worst headache of his life. What might you expect their blood pressure to be?

    Typically this is the description for a subarachnoid hemorrhage. You would expect the blood pressure to be elevated.

- Name one abortive drug for migraines.

    Triptans (sumatriptan, zolmitriptan), ergotamine

- An EEG showing focal rhythmic discharges at the onset of the seizure should make you think of what diagnosis?

    Simple partial seizure

- What is the single most important thing to be concerned about with a patient in status epilepticus?

    Airway, followed by management of hyperthermia

- Describe Brudzinski's sign.

    When you lift the patient's head the patient bends his hips.

NEUROLOGY

Name three medications used to break a seizure?	*Diazepam, lorazepam, phenytoin or fosphenytoin.*
There is an MRI result of multiple foci of demyelination in the white matter. What is the most likely diagnosis?	*Multiple sclerosis*
A patient presents following a seizure. Just before the siezure she remembers seeing flashing lights all around her. What diagnosis should be at the top of your differential?	*Complex partial*
List three medications used to "treat" multiple sclerosis?	*Steroids, interferon beta, copolymer 1*
What is the most common cause of dementia?	*Alzheimer's disease, it may be as high as 80%.*
What four chromosomes have been linked to dementia?	*1,14,19,21*
Is the ankle jerk reflex of lumbar or sacral origin?	*Sacral*
A study result comes back with intracellular neurofibrillary tangles and extracellular neuritic plaques. What is the most likely diagnosis?	*Alzheimer's disease*
A patient complains of an aching headache which feels like a band around his head. What is the most likely diagnosis?	*Tension headache*
A patient presents to your office complaining of a tremor in his right hand. He states after a beer it goes away completely. What is the most likely diagnosis?	*Benign essential tremor or familial tremor*
List two medications you might use to treat an essential tremor.	*Beta blocker (propranolol), primidone*

NEUROLOGY

At what age do symptoms of Huntington's disease appear?	*Around 30 years old*
A 35 year old patient comes to your office because his wife made him. He has been increasingly irritable and moody. She has also noticed that he is very restless. You order a CT scan which shows cerebral atrophy as well as atrophy of the caudate nucleus. What is the most likely diagnosis?	*Huntington's disease*
What is the medication of choice for a patient with Tourette's syndrome?	*Haloperidol*
A slit lamp shows Kayser-Fleischer rings. What is the most likely diagnosis?	*Wilson's disease*
Wilson's disease is associated with a build up of what mineral?	*There is a deficiency of the copper binding protein and therefore a buildup of copper.*
What are the genetic characteristics of Wilson's disease?	*Autosomal recessive, chromosome 13*
What cranial nerve is affected with Bell's palsy?	*CN VII*
A lumbar puncture for a patient with bacterial meningitis will show elevated or decreased WBCs? Glucose? Protein?	*Elevated WBCs, decreased glucose and elevated protein*
What symptom is associated with a classic migraine?	*Having an aura*
Elevated circulating acetylcholine receptor antibodies should make you think of what diagnosis?	*Myasthenia gravis*

NEUROLOGY

☐ Duchenne's and Becker's muscular dystrophy have what genetic characteristic?	*X-linked recessive*
☐ What is the age range for Duchenne's muscular dystrophy?	*3-5 years old*
☐ An EEG showing generalized spikes and associated slow waves should make you think of what diagnosis?	*Generalized or absence seizure*
☐ What is the most common primary intracranial neoplasm?	*Glioma*
☐ What is the most common cause of subarachnoid hemorrhage aside from trauma?	*Ruptured cerebral aneurysm*
☐ What are the most common primary cancer sites that metastasize to the brain?	*Lung, breast and kidney*
☐ A resting or pill-rolling tremor should make you think of what diagnosis?	*Parkinson's disease*
☐ Weakness and numbness in the left hand might be a blockage in which carotid artery?	*Right*
☐ A patient has an intracranial neoplasm causing auditory illusions, olfactory hallucinations and emotional changes. What lobe is the lesion likely in?	*Temporal*
☐ If you are looking for lesions associated with multiple sclerosis and you order an MRI do you order with gadolinium or without?	*With gadolinium*
☐ What is the defining symptom of Alzheimer's?	*Progressive memory impairment*
☐ Which nerve root is responsible for the knee jerk reflex?	*L3-L4*

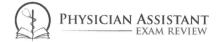

NEUROLOGY

☐ An EEG showing interictal spikes should make you think of what diagnosis?	*Complex partial seizure*
☐ Which is the most commonly herniated vertebral disc?	*L4-L5 followed by L5-S1*
☐ What three symptoms are classic for a normal pressure hydrocephalus?	*Gait disturbance, dementia and urinary incontinence*
☐ A patient presents with inability to speak and right sided weakness. He seems to understand speech and follows commands well. What type of aphasia should you be thinking of?	*Broca's aphasia*
☐ Alcohol may be a major factor in which encephalopathy?	*Wernicke's*
☐ A patient complains of muscle weakness and fatigability that improves with rest. What is the most likely diagnosis?	*Myasthenia gravis*
☐ Lead pipe or cogwheel rigidity should make you think of what diagnosis?	*Parkinson's disease*

PSYCHOLOGY

☐	How long does a panic attack typically last?	*10-20 minutes*
☐	What type of hallucinations are most common in schizophrenia auditory, visual or olfactory?	*Auditory - hearing voices*
☐	What causes anorexic patients to have osteopenia?	*A decrease in estrogen*
☐	When treating psychiatric patients are benzodiazepines used more commonly for acute or chronic treatment?	*Acute*
☐	What is the most common precipitating event for posttraumatic stress disorder in women?	*Rape*
☐	A patient's wife complains that he is hypervigilant and has a hyperstartle response. What is the most likely diagnosis?	*Posttraumatic stress disorder*
☐	Are patients with specific phobias aware they are strange?	*Yes*
☐	A patient complains of having suddenly developed stage fright. It is very important to his career that he be able to speak in front of groups. What medication might you treat him with?	*Beta blocker - propranolol*
☐	A doughnut shaped burn should make you think of what issue?	*Abuse either child or elder*
☐	What is the generic name for Prozac?	*Fluoxetine*
☐	How long must symptoms last before diagnosing ADD?	*6 months*
☐	A patient's mother has recommended that he see you. He lives on his own and is a computer programmer. He works from home. He has no friends and seldom leaves the house. She is concerned that clearly he would like to meet people, but he is terrified of doing so. What is the most likely diagnosis?	*Avoidant personality disorder*

PSYCHOLOGY

- A 6 year old boy seems to have all of the symptoms of ADD while at school, but at home he has no problems. Does he have ADD?

  No, symptoms must occur in both settings for diagnosis.

- An 18 month old is not yet speaking. He does not point to objects. He does not make eye contact with others. What is the most likely diagnosis?

  Autism

- List three positive symptoms of schizophrenia.

  Hallucinations, delusions, movement disorders

- When is the typical onset of Tourette's syndrome?

  3-8 years old

- Is anorexia egosyntonic or ego-dystonic? What about bulimia?

  Anorexia is egosyntonic. Bulimia is ego-dystonic.

- List the three cluster A personality disorders.

  "Mad" schizoid, schizotypal and paranoid

- How long does menstration need to be absent before secondary amenorrhea can be diagnosed?

  If cycles have been previously normal: 3 months. If cycles have been previously irregular: 6 months.

- A 16 year old has just moved schools. He is quiet, moody and not like himself at all. Within six months he seems to have completely changed back to his previous personality. What is the most likely diagnosis?

  Adjustment disorder

- You have a patient with major depressive disorder. Once his symptoms have completely resolved how long should you continue with treatment?

  A six month minimum is recomended due to very high relapse rates.

- What medication is often used to treat postpartum depression in a woman who is breast feeding?

  Sertraline (Zoloft)

- A patient has very strange magical thinking. What is the most likely diagnosis?

  Schizotypal personality disorder

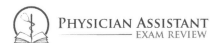

PSYCHOLOGY

List four symptoms of serotonin syndrome.	*Hyperthermia!, seizure, mental status change, tremor*
What is the term for a chronic mild depression which has lasted greater than two years?	*Dysthymia*
What is necessary to diagnose a patient with bipolar 1?	*One manic episode. They do not have to have the depressive episode for the diagnosis.*
What is the major concern with using lithium?	*It has a very narrow therapeutic window. Blood tests are needed every four weeks.*
A patient believes that her 15 year old daughter is sleeping with the mailman. She has no evidence of this. She has confronted her daughter who denies it. It is not interfering with her daily activities, but she does spend time thinking about it. What is the most likely diagnosis?	*Delusional disorder*
At what BMI should a patient be hospitalized for anorexia?	*BMI of <17.5 or 20% below appropriate body weight*
What is the term for being afraid of being out in a terrible situation with no help available?	*Agoraphobia*
Borderline personality disorder is on the border of what two psychological disorders?	*Neurosis and psychosis*
Waxy flexibility should make you think of what diagnosis?	*Catatonic schizophrenia*
How long before normal grief resolves?	*About one year*

PSYCHOLOGY

A patient of yours always craves attention, often using sex as a tool to gain it. She often acts like a child when she does not get her way? What is the most likely diagnosis?	*Histrionic personality disorder*
To be diagnosed with ADD patients must exhibit symptoms before what age?	*7 years old*
What is Russell's sign?	*Abraded knuckles from forcing oneself to vomit.*
How long must symptoms occur before diagnosing schizophrenia?	*At least six months*
Posturing should make you think of what diagnosis?	*Catatonic depression*
A patient complains of acute paralysis in his left arm. This does not seem to bother him, but his wife made him come in. There was no traumatic event. A complete neurologic workup is negative. What is the most likely diagnosis?	*Conversion disorder*
A psychiatric patient presents with confusion, fever and lead pipe rigidity. What is the most likely diagnosis?	*Neuroleptic malignant syndrome, this can occur with high dose antipsychotics.*
A patient is very concerned that she has breast cancer. In order to reassure her you perform a full workup which is negative. She is still unsatisfied and convinced that she has breast cancer. What is the most likely diagnosis?	*Hypochondriasis*
What is the time frame for the first symptoms of withdrawal from alcohol?	*Tremor in 8-18 hrs*
How do you treat alcohol withdrawal?	*Benzodiazepines*

PSYCHOLOGY

- List the four cluster B personality disorders.

    "Bad" antisocial, borderline, histrionic and narcissistic

- List the two cluster C personality disorders.

    "Sad" avoidant and obsessive compulsive

- What medication is clearly contraindicated in anorexia and bulimia?

    Bupropion (Wellbutrin) because it can increase risk of seizures.

- What two psychiatric issues are more common in males than females?

    Autism and ADD, the rest are all either equal or more common in females.

- A patient's mother has recommended that he see you. He lives on his own and is a computer programmer. He works from home. He has no friends and seldom leaves the house. She is concerned that he expresses no interest in meeting people and seems perfectly happy to be home alone all the time. What is the most likely diagnosis?

    Schizoid personality disorder

- Name three SSRI's

    Fluoxetine, paroxetine, sertraline, citalopram, escitalopram, dapoxetine, zimelidine, mesembrine, seproxetine

- A patient expresses concern that he can't trust anyone. That everyone is out to get him, and his problems are all the faults of others. He has held very long grudges due to perceived past wrongs. What is the most likely diagnosis?

    Paranoid personality disorder

- A patient is very charming during his interview. You note during your interview that he has no concern for hurting or using other people. He seems to show no remorse for any of his actions. What is the most likely diagnosis?

    Antisocial personality disorder

- Antisocial personality disorder may not be diagnosed until what age?

    18 years old

PSYCHOLOGY

A patient exhibits all of the characteristics of antisocial personality disorder, but he is only 14 years old. What is the most likely diagnosis?	Conduct disorder
A patient exhibits splitting, seeing others as all good or all bad. What is the most likely diagnosis?	Borderline personality disorder
What type of behavioral therapy works best for borderline patients?	Dialectical behavior therapy
A patient is arrogant with an inflated self image. He feels he is special and should be treated that way. What is the most likely diagnosis?	Narcissistic personality disorder
Is obsessive compulsive disorder egosyntonic or ego-dystonic? What about obsessive compulsive personality disorder?	OCD is ego-dystonic. OCPD is egosyntonic.
What two things are needed to make a diagnosis of bipolar 2?	One major depressive episode and one hypomanic episode
What medication is a good place to start treating bipolar 1 or 2?	Lithium
How is acute stress disorder different than posttraumatic stress disorder?	Acute stress disorder occurs within 1 month of event and resolves within about a month. PTSD begins at about 1 month after event and can last indefinitely.
A spiral fracture should make you think of what issue?	Abuse, either child or elder
During an interview a patient states "I have been anxious for as long as I can remember." This statement should make you think of what diagnosis?	Generalized anxiety disorder
Are hallucinations normal during a normal grieving period?	Yes, as long as they are not persistent or intrusive.

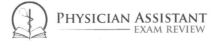

CARDIOLOGY

What side effect might make a patient stop taking an ACEI?	*Cough*
Define orthostatic hypotension.	*A drop in systolic blood pressure of >20 mmhg when standing up.*
You feel a pulse that seems to be vibrating. What term do you use to describe it?	*Thrill*
What are three things in your differential if you have a paradoxical pulse?	*Cardiac tamponade, pericarditis and obstructive lung disease*
On palpation, what size is normal for the aorta?	*Less than 3 cm*
A fixed or consistent split S2 should make you think of what diagnosis?	*Atrial septal defect*
A pathologic S3 is most commonly associated with what diagnosis?	*CHF*
If you hear a midsystolic click you should immediately be thinking about what diagnosis?	*Mitral valve prolapse*
An opening snap on auscultation of the heart should make you think of what diagnosis?	*Mitral stenosis*
A continuous murmur most likely involves what area of the heart?	*It is most likely a septal defect.*
You hear a continuous machine-like murmur. What is the most likely diagnosis?	*Patent ductus arteriosus (PDA)*
List three medications which may be used for pharmacological stress test.	*Adenosine, dobutamine, dipyridamole and persantine*
What is the gold standard for diagnosing coronary artery disease?	*Cardiac catheterization*

CARDIOLOGY

Define stage 1 hypertension according to JNC 7.	*Systolic pressure of 140-159 and diastolic of 90-99*
What is the treatment goal for a diabetic with hypertension?	*130/80*
What is the most common cause of secondary hypertension?	*Chronic kidney disease*
No matter what medications you use you are having trouble keeping a patient's blood pressure under control. You also notice hyperpigmented skin and truncal obesity. What is the most likely diagnosis?	*Cushing's disease*
List three signs or symptoms which will likely be included in a description of a patient with a pheochromocytoma?	*Thin, diaphoretic, tachycardic, agitated and hypertensive*
You have a patient with diagnosis of a pheochromocytoma. While waiting for surgery, should you use an alpha blocker or a beta blocker?	*Alpha blocker. You should never use a pure beta blocker.*
A young boy comes into your office. He has elevated blood pressure when taken in his arm, but no femoral pulses can be palpated. What is the most likely diagnosis?	*Coarctation of the aorta*
According to the CDC, what is the range for a normal BMI?	*18.5-24.9*
What is the first line medical treatment for stage 1 hypertension?	*Thiazide diuretic*
After a thiazide diuretic, what medication should you start in a hypertensive patient who also has diabetes?	*An ACEI or an ARB*

CARDIOLOGY

Following a myocardial infarction, what medication should you be using to treat hypertension?	Beta blocker
Paroxysmal nocturnal dyspnea should make you think of what diagnosis?	CHF
What is the most common cause of CHF?	Coronary artery disease
What ejection fraction is typical for a patient with CHF?	35-40%
What is the most likely diagnosis for a young man who experiences sudden death while playing sports?	Hypertrophic cardiomyopathy
Bat wing vessels or Kerley B lines on a CXR should make you think of what diagnosis?	CHF
A beta natriuretic peptide below what level rules out CHF?	< 100
What is the therapeutic range for INR following a mechanical valve replacement?	2.5-3.5
What is the first line IV inotropic agent when dealing with cardiogenic shock?	Dopamine
What diagnosis is most likely in an IV drug user with a new heart murmur and fever?	Endocarditis
List two diagnoses which require antibiotic prophylaxis for "dirty procedures?"	Prosthetic valve, valve repair with any prosthetic material, prior endocarditis diagnosis, congenital cyanotic heart defect
Does a patient with mitral valve prolapse require prophylactic antibiotics for dental work?	No, a recent change moves mitral valve prolapse from high risk to moderate risk.

CARDIOLOGY

☐ What are the three major criteria for endocarditis?	2 positive blood cultures, a positive transesophageal echocardiography, new murmur
☐ Which are painful and found on the fingers and toes, Osler nodes or Janeway lesions?	Osler nodes
☐ List the 4 minor criteria for diagnosing endocarditis.	Fever, embolic event (Janeway lesions or petechiae, splinter hemorrhages), immunological event (osler nodes, glomerulonephritis), 1 positive blood culture
☐ What are the five components of tetralogy of Fallot?	Ventricular septal defect, right ventricular hypertrophy, right ventricular outflow obstruction (pulmonary valve stenosis), overriding aorta, right sided aortic arch
☐ What is the gold standard for diagnosing myocarditis?	Myocardial biopsy
☐ Where do most aortic dissections occur?	The ascending or descending thoracic aorta
☐ A patient complains of severe pleuritic chest pain that is relieved with sitting and leaning forward. What is the most likely diagnosis?	Pericarditis
☐ What is the first line medical treatment for pericarditis?	Aspirin and NSAIDS
☐ What is the name of the syndrome that involves pericarditis several days after a myocardial infarction?	Dressler syndrome
☐ A patient presents to the ER with chest pain. An EKG shows diffuse ST elevations in almost all of the leads. What is the most likely diagnosis?	Pericarditis

CARDIOLOGY

Define paradoxical pulse.	*There is a large difference in pulse pressure between inhalation and exhalation.*
Define pulsus alternans.	*EKG waveform changes from beat to beat*
What is the definitive treatment for cardiac tamponade?	*Pericardiocentesis*
On physical exam, you hear a harsh systolic murmur along the right sternal border. What is the most likely diagnosis?	*Aortic stenosis*
A wide pulse pressure with a blowing diastolic decrescendo murmur at the right 2nd intercostal space should make you think of what diagnosis?	*Aortic regurgitation*
What is the best location to hear problems with the aortic valve?	*2nd right intercostal space*
Where is disease of the pulmonary valve best heard?	*2nd left intercostal space*
What two antibiotics are used for empiric treatment of endocarditis?	*Vancomycin and ceftriaxone together are first line empiric treatment*
What two valvular issues do patients with Marfan's syndrome often have?	*Aortic regurgitation and mitral valve prolapse (you can tell them apart by where they are heard).*
What are the two main causes of aortic stenosis?	*Congenital bicuspid valve and calcification of the valve secondary to coronary artery disease*
An elderly patient presents with dyspnea, angina and syncope on exertion. The EKG is normal. What is the most likely diagnosis?	*Aortic stenosis*

CARDIOLOGY

- On auscultation, you hear a harsh, blowing, pansystolic murmur at the apex. What is the most likely diagnosis?
  Mitral regurgitation

- You suspect mitral regurgitation. What is the most accurate way to prove your diagnosis?
  Transesophageal echo

- A patient with mitral valve prolapse will often have what physical characteristics?
  Often a thin female

- What is the best patient position to hear aortic regurge and aortic stenosis?
  Sitting up and leaning forward

- What is Tietze syndrome?
  Costochondritis

- Are most pulmonary valve problems congenital or acquired?
  95% are congenital

- What is the therapeutic range for INR following an organic valve replacement?
  2 to 3

- A 60 year old male presents to the ER with severe dizziness and back pain. His blood pressure is dropping, and you can feel an abdominal pulsatile mass on physical exam. What is the most likely diagnosis?
  Ruptured aortic aneurysm

- In a patient with aortic stenosis, will the PMI be medially displaced, normal or laterally displaced?
  It will be laterally displaced due to left ventricular hypertrophy.

- A patient complains of severe crushing chest pain. EKG shows ST segment elevations. All labs including troponins and CK-MB are negative. What is the most likely diagnosis?
  Prinzmetal's angina

- A question about Prinzmetal's angina will often contain what key thing in the patient's history?
  Cocaine use

CARDIOLOGY

- Name two things that would constitute a positive stress test.

  A drop in blood pressure, a new arrhythmia, an increase in angina symptoms, ST depressions

- Are ulcers from venous insufficiency painful or painless?

  Painless

- A patient has just received a cardiac stent. How long will he be on aspirin and clopidogrel?

  One year

- Where is disease of the mitral valve best heard?

  At the apex

- What is the initial treatment for a myocardial infarction?

  MONA - morphine, oxygen, nitroglycerin and aspirin

- Clot busting drugs should be used within 3 hours of which two cardiac events?

  STEMI and new left bundle branch block

- List three catastrophic complications of a myocardial infarction.

  Papillary muscle rupture, myocardial wall rupture and left ventricular aneurysm

- An EKG shows a regular heart rate of 200 bpms. QRS is narrow. What is the most likely diagnosis?

  Supraventricular tachycardia

- Acute endocarditis is most commonly caused by what organism?

  Staph aureus

- List three congenital heart diseases.

  Atrial septal defect (ASD), ventricular septal defect (VSD), coarctation of the aorta, patent ductus arteriosus (PDA), tetralogy of Fallot

- What is the most common cause of an atrial septal defect?

  Patent foramen ovale

- Where on your patient should you listen for the murmur associated with an atrial septal defect?

  At the left second or third interspace

CARDIOLOGY

- A CXR shows a "3" sign with notching of the ribs. What is the most likely diagnosis? — *Coarctation of the aorta*

- What is the appropriate treatment for a patent ductus arteriosus. — *Indomethacin*

- A Blalock procedure is used to correct what congenital heart condition? — *Tetralogy of Fallot*

- You hear a loud, harsh pulmonary murmur along the left sternal border. What is the most likely diagnosis? — *Ventricular septal defect*

- Subacute endocarditis is most commonly caused by what organism? — *Strep Viridans*

- What is the most common place for an aortic aneurysm? — *In the abdomen and below the renal arteries*

- Who is more likely to have an aortic aneurysm males or females? — *Males are eight times as likely to have an aortic aneurysm.*

- The accessory pathway known as the James bundle should make you think of what syndrome? — *Lown-Ganong-Levine syndrome*

- What imaging needs to be done before taking a patient to the OR with an aortic aneurysm? — *CT (echo may be used as initial study, but CT is need for surgery)*

- List two risk factors for an aortic dissection? — *Hypertension, Marfan's syndrome, bicuspid aortic valve, pregnancy*

- A patient presents to the ER with tearing chest pain radiating to his back. What is the most likely diagnosis? — *Aortic dissection*

- What will a CXR show for a patient with an aortic dissection? — *Widened mediastinum*

CARDIOLOGY

What is the best test to diagnose an aortic dissection?	*CT*
List the six P's of an ischemic limb.	*Pain, paresthesias, pallor, pulselessness, poikilothermia, paralysis*
You have a patient with pulsus paradoxus. What two diagnosis should you be thinking of?	*Pericarditis, pericardial effusion and an obstructive lung issue*
A patient complains of pain in his legs when he walks. It goes away after sitting. What term comes to mind for this symptom? What diagnosis is it associated with?	*Intermittent claudication caused by peripheral arterial disease.*
Giant cell arteritis is associated with what other disease?	*Polymyalgia rheumatica*
A sawtooth pattern on EKG should make you think of what diagnosis?	*Atrial flutter*
What is the accessory pathway associated with Wolff-Parkinson-White syndrome?	*The bundle of Kent*
A biphasic P wave should make you think of what diagnosis?	*Left atrial enlargement*
What is the gold standard for diagnosis of giant cell arteritis?	*Biopsy of the temporal artery*
What is the treatment for giant cell arteritis?	*High dose prednisone*
List the components of Virchow's triad.	*Stasis, vascular injury, hypercoagulability*
Calf pain should always make you think of what diagnosis?	*DVT*
Where is disease of the tricuspid valve best heard?	*Along the left lower sternal border*

CARDIOLOGY

What is the most common congenital heart disease?	Ventricular septal defect
Are ulcers from arterial insufficiency painful or painless?	Painful
Give two contraindications for using an ACEI.	Bilateral renal artery stenosis, history of angioedema, pregnancy
Both lead I and AVF have positive QRS complexes. Does this represent normal axis, left axis deviation or right axis deviation?	Normal axis
What medication might you switch to if a patient develops an intolerable cough on an ACEI?	Angiotensin receptor blocker (ARBs)
What class of cardiac medications should be avoided in patients with asthma?	Beta blockers (Blocks receptors for bronchodilators)
A boot-shaped heart on CXR should make you think of what congenital heart condition?	Tetralogy of Fallot
An RSR prime in leads V1 or V2 should make you think of what diagnosis?	Right bundle branch block
Which lab should be tightly monitored in a patient taking an aldosterone antagonist?	Potassium, they may have hyperkalemia.
What is the best test for diagnosing CHF?	Echo
Which cardiac medication is used to help with cardiac contractility after you have optimized most of the other cardiac medications?	Digoxin
A blockage of which artery causes an anterior wall MI?	Left anterior descending artery
What lab result will increase the risk of digoxin toxicity?	Hypokalemia or hypercalcemia

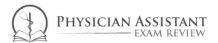

CARDIOLOGY

- A patient presents to the ER in acute CHF. What drug class will likely be the first choice?

  Loop diuretics

- A patient has a GFR of 25 and HTN. Which class should you use, a loop or a thiazide diuretic?

  A loop will work no matter how low the GFR is. Thiazides will only work with a GFR over 30.

- Which EKG leads are used to diagnose an anterior wall MI?

  V1, V2 and V3

- Do loop diuretics cause hyperkalemia or hypokalemia?

  Hypokalemia

- Statins are the drug of choice to treat what type of dyslipidemia?

  Elevated LDL

- A patient recently started taking Lipitor. He is now complaining of aches and pains. What test should you order?

  Serum creatinine kinase, you're looking for rhabdomyolysis.

- How does ezetimibe work?

  Decreases intestinal absorption of cholesterol.

- Which hyperlipidemia medication may cause flushing?

  Niacin

- Name three medication "classes" which are used to reduce LDL?

  Statins, ezetimibe, niacin and nicotinic acid

- Name two fibric acid derivatives.

  Fenofibrate and gemfibrozil

- List three class 1a antiarrhythmics.

  Disopyramide, quinidine, procainamide

- You are counting boxes from the peak of a QRS wave on an EKG in order to determine the heart rate. What would the heart rate be if the next QRS wave peak were three boxes away? What numbers are associated with the first five boxes?

  The answer is 100. The heart rates by counting boxes are 300, 150, 100, 75, 60.

CARDIOLOGY

A U wave on EKG should make you think of what diagnosis?	Hypokalemia
What will the heart rate be if the AV node is pacing the heart?	40-60 beats per minute
Which cardiac medication has gynecomastia in its side effect profile?	Spironolactone
Lead I has a QRS that is up and the AVF lead has a QRS complex that is down. Does this represent normal axis, left axis deviation or right axis deviation?	Left axis deviation
An Osborn or J wave on EKG should make you think of what diagnosis?	Hypothermia
What is the first line medication for a patient with symptomatic bradycardia?	Atropine
What is the heart rate for tachycardia? How about bradycardia?	Tachycardia >100, bradycardia <60
On EKG there is an early but otherwise normal PQRS complex. After that beat there is a slight pause and then a normal rhythm continues. What is the term for this one beat?	Premature atrial contraction
How do you treat polymyalgia rheumatica?	Low dose prednisone
What is the management of a patient in supraventricular tachycardia?	Vagal maneuvers, carotid massage, adenosine
What is the definitive treatment for atrial flutter?	Radiofrequency catheter ablation
An 82 year old patient complains of headaches and jaw claudication. What is the most likely diagnosis?	Giant cell (temporal) arteritis

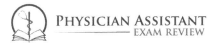

CARDIOLOGY

☐ The EKG shows irregularly irregular narrow QRS waves. What diagnosis should you be thinking of?	*Atrial fibrillation*
☐ An EKG shows a regular rate of 50 beats per minute. The QRS is narrow and there is no visible P wave. What is the most likely diagnosis?	*Junctional rythm*
☐ Name a common cause of a junctional rhythm.	*Digitoxin toxicity*
☐ An EKG shows two premature ventricular contractions. These two QRS waves look very different. What is the term for this?	*Multifocal premature ventricular contractions*
☐ What is the most common cause of sudden cardiac death?	*Ventricular fibrillation*
☐ A patient in the ER has no pulse; but on EKG, there are wide irregular "complexes" which are at an irregular rate. They all appear very different from one another. What is the treatment for this patient?	*He is in ventricular fibrillation. The treatment is defibrillation.*
☐ Tall peaked T waves should make you think of what diagnosis?	*Hyperkalemia*
☐ How do you define 1st degree AV block?	*The PR interval is longer than 0.2 seconds or one block on EKG.*
☐ What is the other term for Mobitz type I?	*Wenckebach*
☐ What is the most important complication of giant cell arteritis?	*Blindness*
☐ What two labs do you want to monitor in a patient on an ACEI?	*Serum creatinine and serum potassium*
☐ The heart rate is irregular, so you can't count boxes between QRS waves to determine heart rate. What is another method you can use to determine rate on an EKG?	*Count QRS waves in a six second strip and multiply by 10 to get beats per minute.*

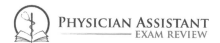

CARDIOLOGY

What is the treatment for a patient with a Mobitz II AV block?	*Pacemaker*
You see regular P waves and regular QRS complexes, but they do not seem to have any correlation to each other. What is the diagnosis?	*Third degree AV block*
Name one aldosterone antagonist.	*Spironolactone, eplerenone*
You see a short PR interval and a delta wave on EKG. What is the most likely diagnosis?	*Wolff-Parkinson-White syndrome*
What two leads do you use to determine the axis of the heart?	*Lead I and AVF*
An RSR prime in leads V5 or V6 should make you think of what diagnosis?	*Left bundle branch block*
Which finding requires immediate attention: left bundle branch block or right bundle branch block?	*New left bundle branch block is a STEMI equivalent. Right bundle branch block is usually not a problem.*
What medication class is used to lower triglycerides?	*Fibric acid derivatives*
Tall peaked P waves should make you think of what diagnosis?	*Right atrial enlargement*
List two causes of right atrial enlargement.	*Pulmonary HTN, severe lung disease, pulmonary valve stenosis*
Which EKG leads are used to diagnose an anterolateral MI?	*V5 and V6*
What are the three inferior leads?	*II, III and aVF*
A blockage of which artery causes a lateral wall MI?	*Left circumflex artery*

CARDIOLOGY

- What is represented by ST segment depressions greater than 1mm on EKG?

    Ischemia

- Rheumatic fever most commonly affects which valve?

    The mitral valve

- What is the only cyanotic congenital heart disease on the NCCPA blueprint?

    Tetralogy of Fallot

- On EKG, there is an early wide QRS complex with no associated P wave. After that beat, there is a slight pause, and then a normal rhythm continues. What is the term for this one beat?

    Premature ventricular contraction

- What is the definitive treatment for a patient with recurrent ventricular tachycardia?

    Implanted defibrillator

- On an EKG, you notice a patient has a gradually lengthening PR interval and then a missed QRS complex. The pattern repeats again. What type of AV block is this?

    Mobitz I or Wenckebach

- List three side effects of digoxin.

    Nausea/vomiting, anorexia, confusion, arrhythmias (sinus brady, AV block), fatigue, vision disturbances etc.

- What is the first line medical treatment for torsades de pointes?

    Magnesium sulfate

DERMATOLOGY

Why should actinic keratosis be treated?	It may progress to squamous cell carcinoma.
What is first line treatment for rosacea?	Metronidazole, tetracycline is probably a close second.
Where are 90% of basal cell lesions found on the body?	On the head and neck
Purple, pruritic, polygonal, papules on physical exam should make you think of what diagnosis?	Lichen planus
What are the ABC's of melanoma?	Asymmetry, border, color, diameter, elevation/irregularity, evolving
A positive Auspitz sign should make you think of what diagnosis?	Psoriasis
What is the key indicator for the prognosis of melanoma?	Thickness of the lesion
What is the treatment for melanoma?	Wide local excision
A waxy stuck on appearance should make you think of what diagnosis?	Seborrheic keratosis
A 5 year old presents in early January with a red itchy rash behind his knees. You notice it on the flexor surfaces of his elbows as well. What is the most likely diagnosis?	Atopic dermatitis
The term satellite lesion should make you think of what diagnosis?	Candida diaper rash
Coin-shaped plaques should make you think of what diagnosis?	Nummular eczema

DERMATOLOGY

☐ A 30 year old female presents with pustules on her face that spare the vermilion border. In her history she has been using topical steroids. What is the most likely diagnosis?	*Perioral dermatitis*
☐ A patient presents with flaky skin in the nasolabial folds and in her hair. What is the most likely diagnosis?	*Seborrheic dermatitis*
☐ How do you treat a stasis dermatitis?	*Compression stockings*
☐ Tapioca blisters should make you think of what diagnosis?	*Dyshidrosis - these are usually on the hands and feet*
☐ How do you treat dyshidrosis?	*Topical steroids*
☐ Giant cells on a Tzanck smear should make you think of what diagnosis?	*Herpes simplex virus*
☐ How do you treat lichen simplex chronicus?	*Get the patient to stop scratching it.*
☐ A herald patch should make you think of what diagnosis?	*Pityriasis rosea*
☐ How do you treat pityriasis rosea?	*Reassurance*
☐ A patient with a history of herpes now presents with a target lesion. What is the most likely diagnosis?	*Erythema multiforme*
☐ Rhinophyma should make you think of what diagnosis?	*Acne rosacea*
☐ Silvery scales should make you think of what diagnosis?	*Psoriasis*
☐ A teardrop lesion after a course of strep throat should make you think of what diagnosis?	*Guttate psoriasis*

DERMATOLOGY

- Are lesions from psoriasis typically found on flexor or extensor surfaces?

    Extensor

- What is the first line treatment for tinea corporis?

    Topical azoles

- What are the two most common organisms responsible for cellulitis?

    Strep and Staph

- Pitting nails are associated with what dermatologic disorder?

    Psoriasis

- Nummular eczema is most like what other dermatological disorder?

    Atopic dermatitis

- Honey-colored crusts should make you think of what diagnosis?

    Impetigo

- What two human papillomaviruses are most responsible for condyloma acuminata?

    HPV 6 and 11

- A double comedone is indicative of what diagnosis?

    Hidradenitis suppurativa

- What is the best treatment for molluscum contagiosum?

    It is self limiting, but can be removed if patient really wants it.

- What is the treatment for seborrheic keratosis?

    It is bengin so there is no need to treat it. Lesions may be removed if unsightly.

- Hyperpigmented velvety plaques should make you think of what diagnosis?

    Acanthosis nigricans

- Melasma is most often found in what patient population?

    Women of childbearing age

- Extremely pruritic lesions with burrows in runs should make you think of what diagnosis?

    Scabies

DERMATOLOGY

What is the first step in treating atopic dermatitis?	*Behavioral modifications - reduce bathing, only use soap on face and genitals, use natural breathable fabrics*
What is the treatment for a bad brown recluse spider bite?	*Debridement, the venom causes tissue necrosis.*
Salmon-colored scales should make you think of what diagnosis?	*Psoriasis*
Depigmented patches of skin should make you think of what diagnosis?	*Vitiligo*
Spaghetti and meatballs on KOH prep should make you think of what diagnosis?	*Tinea versicolor*
What dermatologic finding is associated with insulin insensitivity?	*Acanthosis nigricans*
A slowly growing nodule with a central depression and a pearly border should make you think of what diagnosis?	*Basal cell carcinoma*
What dermatologic finding is associated with asthma?	*Atopic dermatitis*
A christmas tree pattern should make you think of what diagnosis?	*Pityriasis rosea*
Oval patches of hair loss should make you think of what diagnosis?	*Alopecia areata*
What is the first line treatment for genital warts?	*Imiquimod (Aldara)*
A pearly dome-shaped lesion with a central umbilication should make you think of what diagnosis?	*Molluscum contagiousum*
What is the best lab test for scabies?	*Microscopic examination under oil immersion*

ENDOCRINOLOGY

What two hormones are secreted by the posterior pituitary?	Oxytocin and antidiuretic hormone (ADH, vasopressin)
What is Sheehan's syndrome?	Ischemia of the pituitary due to volume depletion during or after childbirth.
How do glitazones work?	They improve insulin sensitivity.
What is the most common pituitary adenoma?	Prolactinoma
Large doughy hands should make you think of what diagnosis?	Gigantism
Diabetes insipidus is caused by a deficiency of which hormone?	Vasopressin
How much more potent is T3 than T4?	3-4x
What is the first line medical treatment for a pheochromocytoma?	Alpha blocker. You should never use a pure beta blocker.
What is the best imaging for a thyroid nodule?	Ultrasound
A patient presents with erectile dysfunction and complains of some numbness in his feet. On second thought he has noticed significant polyuria and polydipsia. What diagnosis should you be thinking of?	Diabetic neuropathy
Pretibial myxedema should make you think of what diagnosis?	Graves' disease
A 35 year old female presents with heat intolerance, weight loss and palpitations. What is the most likely diagnosis?	Hyperthyroidism

ENDOCRINOLOGY

What is the first line medical treatment for a patient who presents with palpitations and nervousness secondary to hyperthyroidism?	Beta Blockers
What is Hashimoto's disease?	An autoimmune cause of hypothyroid
How does levothyroxine work?	It is a synthetic T4
What is the most common thyroid cancer?	Papillary, makes up about 80% of thyroid cancers.
In a patient with hyperthyroidism will TSH most likely be elevated or decreased?	Decreased
How do fibrates work to affect the lipid profile?	They inhibit synthesis of VLDL and elevate lipoprotein lipase.
What medication might you use prior to thyroidectomy in a patient with hyperthyroidism?	Methimazole or propylthiouracil (PTU)
What is included in Whipple's triad of hypoglycemia?	History of previous hypoglycemia, serum glucose of <40, immediate recovery upon administration of glucose
Positive antithyroid peroxidase and antithyroglobulin antibodies should make you think of what diagnosis?	Hashimoto's
What is the treatment for myxedema?	Levothyroxine and slow warming
What is the most common cause of hypoparathyroid?	Post thyroidectomy with the complication of parathyroidectomy.
What is Chvostek's sign?	Tap on facial nerve and get a twitch with low Ca.
Cortical adrenal insufficiency is also known as what disease?	Addison's disease

ENDOCRINOLOGY

What is Trousseau's sign?

Inflate BP cuff and hold for 3 minutes. Patient with low Ca will get carpel tunnel symptoms.

What is the most common cause of hyperparathyroidism?

Single parathyroid adenoma in 80% of cases.

In Cushing's disease is ACTH elevated or decreased?

Elevated

What is Graves' disease?

The most common cause of hyperthyroidism. It is an autoimmune disease.

What specific breathing pattern is associated with diabetic ketoacidosis?

Kussmaul respirations

What is the least aggressive thyroid cancer?

Papillary

Name two tests you might use to rule out Cushing's syndrome.

24 hour free cortisol urine test and dexamethasone suppression test

List two ectopic tumors that may produce ACTH and give a patient Cushing's syndrome?

Small cell lung cancer, pancreatic islet cells, thymomas

What is the treatment for Addison's disease?

Hydrocortisone or prednisone

What is the test to begin with if you suspect a pheochromocytoma?

24 hour urine for catecholamines

Exophthalmos should make you think of what diagnosis?

Hyperthyroidism

What percentage of diabetes in the US is type 2?

80-90%

HLA-DR gene is a marker for what endocrine disorder?

DM type 1

ENDOCRINOLOGY

- What is the main function of parathyroid hormone?

    Increase serum Ca

- List four diagnostic criteria for diabetes?

    Random glucose >200, fasting glucose >126, two hour postprandial glucose >200, HgA1c >6.5%

- Moans, groans, stones and bones describe symptoms of what endocrine problem?

    Hyperparathyroid

- Stocking glove anesthesia should make you think of what diagnosis?

    Diabetic neuropathy and B12 deficiency neuropathy

- Fruity breath should make you think of what diagnosis?

    Diabetic ketoacidosis

- As it relates to diabetics, what is the dawn phenomenon?

    Reduced insulin response between 5 and 8 am

- What is the most common cause of hypopituitarism?

    Tumor

- How does metformin work?

    Decreases the hepatic glucose production and increases peripheral glucose uptake

- How do sulfonylureas work?

    They stimulate the production of insulin.

- What class of medications does pioglitazone (Actos) fall into?

    Thiazolidinediones also known as glitazones

- What is the suffix associated with sulfonylureas?

    Ide is the suffix. Examples: glipizide, tolbutamide, tolazamide.

- Typically what is the first medication started in type 2 DM?

    Metformin

ENDOCRINOLOGY

How often should a diabetic's HgbA1c be checked and what should it be?	*Every three months (remember the life of an RBC is 90-120 days) and it should be below 6.5%*
What are the 5 criteria for metabolic syndrome?	*HDL <40 men <50 females, BP >135/85, Triglycerides >150, Fasting glucose >100, Waist >40 inches in men >35 inches in women*
What class of medications is the first line for lowering LDL?	*Statins*
Which lipid medication may cause flushing?	*Niacin*
What life threatening side effect do statins have?	*Rhabdomyolysis*
Does niacin increase or decrease HDL?	*Increase*
What medication class does metformin (Glucophage) fall into?	*Biguanide*
List the 5 insulins in order of peak efficacy?	*Lispro 1-2 hrs, Regular 2-4 hrs, NPH 5-7 hrs, Lente 4-8 hrs, Ultralente 8-14 hrs*
Is metformin indicated or contraindicated in renal failure?	*Contraindicated*
What is the most common cause of DM type 1?	*Autoimmune destruction of the islet cells in the pancreas*
List 4 physical exam findings for Cushing's syndrome.	*Moon face, buffalo hump, purple striae, central obesity, supraclavicular fat pads, easy bruising*
Propranolol belongs to what class of medication?	*Beta blockers*
During pregnancy which is the prefered treatment of hyperthyroidism PTU or methimazole?	*PTU*

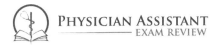

ENDOCRINOLOGY

Name the four thyroid cancers.	*Papillary, Follicular, Medullary, Anaplastic*
What heparin complication is relevant to endocrinology?	*Adrenal infarct leading to a Cushing's syndrome*
How does nicotinic acid work to affect the lipid profile?	*It inhibits secretion of VLDL.*
Hyperpigmentation of the skin along creases should make you think of what diagnosis?	*Addison's disease*
Which thyroid cancer is the most aggressive?	*Anaplastic*
How do statins work to affect the lipid profile?	*They slow the rate limiting step of cholesterol synthesis.*
Will ACTH be elevated or decreased in Addison's disease?	*Elevated if the problem is at the adrenal glands.*
What role does C-peptide play in the diagnosis of diabetes?	*It is a marker of insulin production. Elevated C-peptide points to DM 2. Decreased C-peptide points towards DM 1.*

ENT

- Acute sinusitis is most commonly caused by which two pathogens?

    Strep pneumoniae and haemophilus influenzae

- Oral herpes is best treated with systemic or topical antivirals?

    Topical is the first line. Systemic antivirals will help but are only indicated for severe cases.

- A patient presents with several episodes of vertigo over the past few weeks. He has had intermittent unilateral hearing loss and a "blowing" in his ears. What is the most likely diagnosis?

    Meniere's disease

- A white oral lesion which cannot be scraped off should make you think of what diagnosis?

    Oral leukoplakia

- What type of hearing loss is associated with aging?

    Sensory

- Which is the most commonly affected sinus in acute sinusitis?

    Maxillary

- A patient presents with a hot potato or muffled voice. What is the most likely diagnosis?

    Peritonsillar abscess

- What time frame are we talking about for chronic sinusitis?

    >3 months

- List the time of year when each of the following allergens is most prominent: pollen, grass, mold and ragweed.

    Pollen from trees and flowers = spring, grasses are the summer, mold and ragweed are fall

- How long should pressure be applied to treat epistaxis?

    15 minutes

- List the four things that suggest group A beta-hemolytic strep in a patient with pharyngitis.

    Fever, tender anterior cervical adenopathy, no cough and an exudate in the throat

- A child presenting with an erythematous sandpaper rash should make you think of what diagnosis?

    Scarlet fever

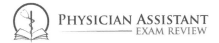

ENT

- In a patient with sensorineural hearing loss, what will be the results of the Weber test?

    The patient will hear the sound louder in the unaffected ear.

- List four complications of untreated strep throat.

    Scarlet fever, glomerulonephritis, rheumatic fever and local abscess

- A patient presents with a round ulcer in her mouth that is yellow-grey and has a red halo. It is on the buccal mucosa and it is painful. What is the most likely diagnosis?

    Aphthous ulcers

- A patient presents drooling, with stridor and in tripod position. What is the diagnosis, and how do you treat it?

    You treat epiglottitis with a second or third generation cephalosporin like cefuroxime or ceftriaxone.

- White oral lesions which can be scraped off leaving punctate bleeding should make you think of what diagnosis?

    Oral candida

- What are three possible treatments for peritonsillar abscess?

    Needle aspiration, I&D and tonsillectomy

- What virus causes mumps?

    Paramyxovirus

- How do you treat allergic rhinitis?

    Intranasal corticosteroid and antihistamines

- What is the treatment of choice for strep throat?

    Penicllin, amoxicillin, erythromycin

- A patient presents with unilateral hearing loss and a decrease in speech discrimination. She has also had difficulty with balance over the past week. What is the most likely diagnosis?

    Acoustic neuroma

- A patient presents with acute swelling and pain in the cheek that increases at meals. What is the most likely diagnosis?

    Sialadenitis (salivary gland infection) - Staph aureus

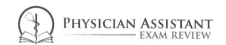

ENT

When is watchful waiting with a diagnosis of acoustic neuroma an appropriate plan?	This tumor is very slow growing. Watching a small tumor in an elderly patient is appropriate treatment.
What type of hearing loss would be caused by cerumen impaction?	Conductive
How do you administer the Weber hearing test?	Tuning fork placed in the middle of the forehead
A 14 year old field hockey player presents with prominent adenopathy, white purple exudates in the throat and a palpable spleen. What is the most likely diagnosis?	Mononucleosis
How do you administer the Rinne hearing test?	Place the tuning fork on the mastoid and then move it next to the ear.
Describe the result of a Weber hearing test in a patient with conductive hearing loss.	Patient will report the sound louder in the affected ear.
An x-ray of the skull reveals coalescence of mastoid air cells. What is the most likely diagnosis?	Mastoiditis
After 7 days of sinusitis what antibiotic would you start?	Amoxicillin or Bactrim
A 45 year old female complains of feeling the ground rolling under her feet at times. What is the most likely diagnosis?	Vertigo
A patient with a history of smoking presents with a new onset hoarseness. This has been persistant for the past two weeks. What is the most likely diagnosis?	Laryngeal squamous cell carcinoma

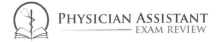

ENT

- A patient presents with acute onset of continuous severe vertigo for the past five days. He does have a history of URI 2 weeks ago. What is the most likely diagnosis?

    Labrynthitis

- What does Kiesselbach's plexus refer to?

    A group of vein's in the anterior nose which bleed a lot

- Small grouped vesicles on the vermillion border should make you think of what diagnosis?

    Herpes

GENITOURINARY

What is the most common type of kidney stone?	*Calcium makes up 85% of kidney stones.*
What is the most specific imaging modality for diagnosing kidney stones?	*CT*
Will a spermatocele transillumnate?	*Yes*
A kidney stone of less than what size will likely pass on its own?	*Less than 5 mm*
List three possible treatments for stress incontinence in women.	*Kegels, estrogen therapy, surgical placement of a urethral sling*
A 65 year old male presents with frequency. On digital rectal exam you feel an elastic moderately enlarged prostate. What is the most likely diagnosis?	*BPH*
A PSA above what level should start to make you concerned?	*>4.0*
Give two major risk factors for erectile dysfunction.	*Diabetes, hypertension, depression, coronary artery disease*
List one major risk factor for bladder cancer?	*Smoking*
Define paraphimosis	*Foreskin is retracted and cannot be reduced.*
Which problem is an emergency phimosis or paraphimosis?	*Paraphimosis*
What is the name of the condition that involves fibrous scar tissue in the penis causing a curvature of the erect penis?	*Peyronie's disease*
Both testicles should be descended by what age?	*3 months*

GENITOURINARY

- [ ] Feeling a bag of worms in the scrotum should make you think of what diagnosis?

    Varicocele

- [ ] A fluid filled painless mass found in the scrotum which transilluminates should make you think of what diagnosis?

    Hydrocele

- [ ] What is the first line treatment for a varicocele?

    Watchful waiting unless there is a question of fertility.

- [ ] Name the sign which is defined as decreased pain with scrotal elevation?

    Prehn's sign

- [ ] Maltese crosses in the urine should make you think of what diagnosis?

    Nephrotic syndrome

- [ ] What is the imaging study of choice if you suspect bladder cancer?

    Cystoscopy and biopsy

- [ ] What is the most likely diagnosis for a free floating, painless, cystic mass found posterior and superior to the testis?

    Spermatocele

- [ ] What age range is typically associated with testicular torsion?

    10-20 years old

- [ ] Where is the epididymis found?

    It is found at the posterior upper pole.

- [ ] What is the best imaging to rule out testicular torsion?

    Doppler U/S for decreased blood flow to the testes

- [ ] What are the two most common causes of epididymitis?

    Neisseria gonorrhea and chlamydia

- [ ] What medicaton classes are prescribed in order to help prevent chronic renal failure in diabetic patients?

    ACEIs or ARBs

GENITOURINARY

Will epididymitis feel better with scrotal elevation?	Yes
What is the normal level of serum bicarbonate (HCO3)?	24 mEq/Liter
What is the treatment for epididymitis?	Ceftriaxone and doxycycline
What is the first line antibiotic treatment for cystitis?	Bactrim
What is the most common organism that causes a bladder infection?	E. coli
Tenderness at the costovertebral angle should make you think of what diagnosis?	Pyelonephritis
What is the condition where the urethral meatus is not at the tip of the penis?	Hypospadias and in far fewer cases epispadias
What is the most common organism responsible for prostatitis?	E. coli
What is the first line antibiotic for prostatitis?	Bactrim 4-6 weeks
List two risk factors for prostate cancer.	Advancing age, African American, positive family history, high fat diet
What might you feel on a digital rectal exam of a patient with prostate cancer?	Enlarged prostate, hard nodules within the prostate
Define priapism	Painful persistent erection
A prostate biopsy consists of how many samples?	6 to 12
Painless hematuria should make you think of what diagnosis?	Bladder cancer
What is the most common bladder cancer?	Transitional cell cancer

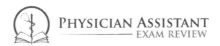

GENITOURINARY

- Define phimosis. — *Foreskin can not be retracted.*

- Name the condition in which the head of the penis curves downward or upward, at the junction of the head and shaft of the penis. (Hint: It is often associated with hypospadias.) — *Chordee*

- How do you treat urethritis? — *Ceftriaxone and doxycycline*

- A 3 year old boy presents with hematuria and a painless palpable abdominal mass. What is the most likely diagnosis? — *Wilms tumor*

- List three possible causes of prerenal renal failure. — *CHF, severe dehydration, hemorrhage*

- What is the most common cause of postrenal renal failure? — *BPH, postrenal renal failure is secondary to an outflow obstruction*

- Muddy-brown sediment in the urine should make you think of what diagnosis? — *Acute tubular necrosis*

- Tea-colored urine with red cell casts should make you think of what diagnosis? — *Glomerulonephritis*

- What are the two most common predisposing factors in the development of chronic renal failure? — *HTN and DM*

- A sponge-like prostate on digital rectal exam should make you think of what diagnosis? — *Prostatitis, but be careful. You can cause sepsis with a digital rectal exam.*

- Will serum potassium be decreased or elevated in renal failure? — *Elevated*

- A urine protein of >3.5 grams/day should make you think of what diagnosis? — *Nephrotic syndrome*

- What hereditary pattern does polycystic kidney disease follow? — *Autosomal dominant*

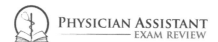

GENITOURINARY

What is the normal pH of the blood?	7.35-7.45
What is the most accurate way to diagnose urethritis?	Urine PCR
What is considered a normal PCO2?	40mmHG
An ABG shows a pH of 7.2, a bicarb of 25 and a PCO2 of 50. Is this respiratory or metabolic acidosis?	Respiratory - CO2 is elevated
White blood cell casts should make you think of what diagnosis?	Pyelonephritis
What area of the prostate is affected by BPH?	The transitional zone
What area of the prostate is the primary site for prostate cancer?	The peripheral zone
An involuntary loss of urine during coughing or laughing is what type of incontinence?	Stress incontinence
A patient who has normal bladder function, but can not get to the bathroom has what type of incontinence?	Functional incontinence
What type of incontinence is often associated with BPH?	Overflow incontinence, the bladder cannot empty sufficiently
At what age do you begin screening patients for prostate cancer? What two tests are used?	At age 50 an annual digital rectal exam and a PSA are recommended.
Often caused by chlamydia what is the syndrome characterized by urethritis (or cervicitis), arthritis and conjuctivitis?	Reiter's syndrome
What is the most common type of testicular cancer?	Nonseminoma

HEMATOLOGY

- What is the normal range for MCV? — *80-100*

- What is the most common microcytic anemia? — *Iron deficiency anemia*

- Would anemia of chronic disease most likely be macrocytic, normocytic or microcytic? — *Normocytic*

- What two main causes should you be thinking of in a macrocytic anemia? — *Malnutrition and severe blood loss*

- Does an increase in reticulocytes indicate a decrease or an increase in RBC production? — *An increase, reticulocytes are newly released "baby" RBC's*

- Auer rods are most commonly associated with what disease? — *Acute myeloid leukemia*

- What molecule binds iron in the blood stream? — *Transferrin*

- What does koilonychia refer to? — *Spoon-shaped nails which may be found in microcytic anemia.*

- Will the serum ferritin be high or low in a patient with iron deficient anemia? — *It will almost always be low.*

- A low retic count and a normal serum ferritin should make you think of what diagnosis? — *Anemia of chronic disease*

- Under normal conditions at what hemoglobin level would you begin to consider a transfusion? — *8*

- Asplenism secondary to sickle cell disease increases a patient's risk for what type of infections? — *Capsulated organisms like Strep pneumo and H. flu*

- An African American teenager presents with avascular necrosis of the his right femoral head. What is the most likely diagnosis? — *Sickle cell disease*

HEMATOLOGY

How do you treat a sickle cell crisis?	Fluids, oxygen, pain medication, transfusion may be necessary
Will unconjugated bilirubin be high or low in a patient with sickle cell disease?	High
Which anemia should you think of if you see the term Howell-Jolly bodies?	Sickle cell due to the functional asplenia, but it may also show up in folic acid deficiency.
G6PD deficiency follows what pattern of inheritance?	X-linked
List the three diagnosis you should be thinking of if a question includes Heinz bodies.	G6PD deficiency anemia, chronic liver disease, alpha thalassemia
What is pica?	Eating non-food items including ice, paper, dirt, hair.
Are target cells seen in mild or severe iron deficiency anemia?	Severe, they are also seen in alpha thalassemia, chronic liver disease and asplenia.
Iron deficiency anemia will have a serum iron lower than what value?	30
Would a B12 deficiency anemia most likely be microcytic, normocytic or macrocytic?	Macrocytic
You should be thinking alpha thalassemia if the question stem includes which four geographic areas?	Southeast Asia, China, Middle East, Africa
A patient of Mediterranean descent is a clue for which type of anemia?	Beta thalassemia
In a folic acid deficiency anemia the folic acid level is typically below what level?	<150

HEMATOLOGY

- What hematological disorder should you think of if the questions talks about the patient eating ice or dirt?

    Iron deficiency anemia

- Inability to absorb vitamin B12 due to lack of intrinsic factor is what disease?

    Pernicious anemia

- Stocking glove paresthesias should make you think of what two diagnoses?

    B12 deficiency neuropathy and diabetic neuropathy

- Will the RBC's be large, small or normal size in a B12 deficient anemia?

    Macrocytes

- Will the retic count be elevated, decreased or normal in a B12 deficient anemia?

    Retic count will be low. Low building blocks means low production.

- What is Schilling's test used for?

    Test for the cause of a B12 deficiency.

- Strict vegans are at risk for what type of anemia?

    B12 deficiency anemia

- Is sickle cell microcytic, macrocytic or normocytic?

    Microcytic

- Will a hemolytic anemia generally have an elevated or decreased retic count?

    Elevated

- List four disease states in which you may find basophilic stippling.

    Lead poisoning, beta or alpha thalassemia, sideroblastic anemia, arsenic poisoning

- If a question presents a pregnant woman with anemia what is the most likely diagnosis?

    Iron deficiency

- The term Philadelphia chromosome should make you think of what diagnosis?

    Chronic myeloid leukemia

INFECTIOUS DISEASE

- White curd like vaginal discharge should make you think of what diagnosis?

  Vaginal candida infection

- Owl eye inclusion bodies should make you think of what diagnosis?

  Cytomegalovirus (CMV)

- If you have a patient with positive blood cultures for candida what is the first line drug?

  Amphotericin B

- What is the treatment for pertussis?

  Erythromycin x 7 days

- A leukemia patient has a CT of the liver which shows punched out lesions. What diagnosis should you be thinking of?

  Hepatosplenic candida

- What disease does Rickettsia rickettsii cause?

  Rocky Mountain spotted fever

- An India ink stain showing cysts should make you think of what diagnosis?

  Cryptococcosis

- A COPD patient has apical cavities and calcified nodes on his CXR. You also discover he has a pet bat and a few birds. What is the most likely diagnosis?

  Histoplasmosis

- An HIV patient presents with a nonproductive cough and a CXR showing diffuse interstitial infiltrates. What is the most likely diagnosis?

  Pneumocystis jiroveci pneumonia (PCJ) formerly known as Pneumocystis pneumonia (PCP)

- Honey and babies should make you think of what diagnosis?

  Botulism

- What type of organism causes botulism?

  A Gram + rod, Clostridium botulinum

- What is the treatment for botulism?

  Antitoxin

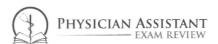

INFECTIOUS DISEASE

- A patient presents to the ER with acute progessive weakness, diplopia and a very dry mouth. What organism may be causing this?

    Clostridium botulinum

- Rice water stool should make you think of what diagnosis?

    Cholera

- Is diphtheria a Gram-positive or negative organism?

    Gram-positive

- A stuck on grey membrane in the pharynx should make you think of what diagnosis?

    Diphtheria

- What are four steps in treating diphtheria?

    Antitoxin, penicillin, remove membrane, report the case to the CDC

- What is the clinical name for whooping cough?

    Pertussis

- What type of organism causes tetanus?

    A Gram + rod, Clostridium tetani

- A patient ate out last night and today has cramping and bloody diarrhea. What is the most likely organism?

    Salmonella

- Diarrhea with blood and mucus should make you think of what diagnosis?

    Shigella

- What is the best test to diagnose malaria?

    Peripheral blood smear

- What organism has been linked to reactive arthritis?

    Shigella, also remember that reactive arthritis has a positive HLA-B27.

- What is the treatment for Shigella?

    Bactrim or fluoroquinolones and hydration.

- What organism causes Lyme disease?

    Borrelia burgdorferi

INFECTIOUS DISEASE

What is the minimum amount of time needed for a tick to transfer Lyme disease to a human?	24 hours
What is the drug of choice to treat Lyme disease in kids or pregnant women?	Amoxicillin
What is the drug of choice to treat C. difficile?	Metronidazole (Flagyl)
A patient was in the woods yesterday and today presents with erythema migrans. What is the most likely diagnosis?	Lyme disease
What drug is used for the treatment or prophylaxis of malaria?	Chloroquine
A patient was camping a few days ago and now has a rash that began on his wrists and ankles. What is the most likely diagnosis?	Rocky Mountain spotted fever
What is the drug of choice for treating Rocky Mountain spotted fever?	Doxycycline
What is the drug of choice for the treatment of syphilis?	Pencillin
Any reference to dark field microscopy should make you think of what organism?	Treponema pallidum
Is staph gram (+) or gram (-)?	Gram (+)
A patient being treated with penicillin for a syphilis infection develops fever, chills, muscle pain and headaches. Do you stop treatment?	No this is Jarisch-Herxheimer reaction. The patient must be closely monitored, but it is a response to released endotoxin from the death of the spirochetes and not an allergic reaction.

INFECTIOUS DISEASE

What organism is believed to be the main culprit in creating peptic ulcers?	*Helicobacter pylori*
A painless, clean base chancre should make you think of what diagnosis?	*Primary syphilis*
Is pseudomonas gram (+) or gram (-)?	*Gram (-)*
A patient complains of a rash on his palms and soles. He has a fever and chills. In conversation he mentions a strange painless chancre he had a few weeks ago. What is the most likely diagnosis?	*Secondary syphilis. This is the most contagious stage.*
What is the treatment for cholera?	*Fluids*
What is the current drug of choice for the cytomegalovirus?	*Ganciclovir*
Which herpesvirus causes Epstein–Barr?	*Herpes 4*
A 16 year old girl presents with an exudative sore throat and general malaise. On physical exam you observe some posterior chain lymphadenopathy and mild splenomegaly. What is the most likely diagnosis?	*Epstein–Barr virus*
What are the two important peices of patient education for anyone diagnosed with mononucleosis?	*No contact sports (splenic rupture) and no kissing (highly contagious)*
What is the first symptom of a rabies infection?	*Pain and anesthesia at the site of the bite*
How do you definitively diagnose rabies?	*Pathology of the brain of the animal that performed the bite using fluorescent antibody stain.*
A patient is bitten by a rabies infected raccoon. On what days do you give human diploid cells?	*0, 3, 7, 14, 28*

INFECTIOUS DISEASE

A diaper rash with satellite lesions should make you think of what diagnosis?	Candida
Name three serious reactions a patient may have with the use of vancomycin?	Nephrotoxicity, ototoxicity and Stevens-Johnson syndrome
What tests are done to screen for HIV?	ELISA and then if the positive diagnosis is confirmed with a Western blot test
What is the drug of choice for the treatment of Lyme disease?	Doxycicline
What does trismus mean?	Lock jaw, often secondary to tetanus
How do you treat amebiasis?	Metronidazole (Flagyl)
How do you treat pneumocystis jiroveci pneumonia (PCJ) formerly known as pneumocystis pneumonia (PCP)?	Bactrim
What is the treatment for a tetanus infections?	Penicillin, immune globulin and supportive care (especially respiratory support)
How do hookworm larvae enter the body?	They penetrate the skin usually through the soles of the feet.
How do you treat hookworm?	Azoles
What type of mosquitoes carry malaria?	Anopheles
How do you treat white oral plaques that can be scraped off?	This is most likely candida. Topical nystatin or oral fluconazole 1 mg are first line choices.
A CT scan shows ring enhancing lesions in an HIV patient. What is the most likely diagnosis?	Toxoplasmosis

INFECTIOUS DISEASE

What is the drug of choice for toxoplasmosis?	Bactrim
What organism causes toxoplasmosis?	Toxoplasma gondii
What drug do you use to treat pinworm?	You treat everyone in the house with albendazole. Two weeks later you treat them again.
The scotch tape test is used to diagnose what disease?	Pinworm
Is neisseria gram (+) or gram (-)?	Gram (-)
Syphilis is caused by what organism?	Treponema pallidum
A Gram-positive organism in chains should make you think of what diagnosis?	Strep
A Gram-negative diplococci should make you think of what diagnosis?	Neisseria
What is the most common prophylactic antibiotic used preoperatively?	Cefazolin = Ancef, Keflex = Cefalexin, The answer is Cefazolin (Ancef)
What oral antibiotic can be used for pseudomonas?	Ciprofloxacin
What is the suffix used for most fluoroquinolones?	Oxacin
Why aren't fluoroquinolones used more frequently?	They have lots of side effects.
A patient presents with a ruptured Achilles tendon. He states he that he was recently in the hospital for a "blood infection and on a ton of antibiotics." What antibiotic class may he have been on?	Fluoroquinolones
Why can't you give fluoroquinolones to kids?	They can cause cartilage development problems.

INFECTIOUS DISEASE

- What class of antibiotics should you start with for community acquired pneumonia?
  Macrolides

- List two macrolides.
  Erythromycin, azithromycin, clarithromycin

- What antibiotic class is the class of choice for chlamydia?
  Macrolides

- What class of antibiotics is sometimes prescribed specifically for its effects on increasing GI motility?
  Macrolides

- Which medication is worse to give to a pediatric patient, tetracycline or an aminoglycoside?
  Tetracycline

- Pizza pie retinopathy should make you think of what diagnosis?
  Cytomegalovirus (CMV)

- A patient presents complaining of a metallic taste in her mouth and dark brown urine. What antibiotic might she be on?
  Metronidazole (Fagyl)

- What antibiotic is most likely to cause C. diff?
  Clindamycin

- What is the current drug of choice for treating MRSA?
  Vancomycin

- You place a patient on rifampin. What side effect should you warn her about?
  Orange-red discoloration of body fluids

- What might happen if you infuse vancomycin too fast?
  Red Man syndrome

- Name one oral medication that can be used for MRSA.
  Linezolid (Zyvox) and Bactrim

- What organism is most commonly responsible for community acquired pneumonia?
  Strep pneumoniae

INFECTIOUS DISEASE

- What organism is the most common cause of an uncomplicated urinary tract infection?

    E. Coli

- Gummas or granulomatous nodules should make you think of what diagnosis?

    Tertiary syphilis

- Bloody stool with cysts and trophozoites should make you think of what diagnosis?

    Amebiasis

- Community acquired carditis is most often caused by one of the HACEK organisms. List the HACEK organisms.

    Haemophilus, Actinobacillus, Cardiobacterium, Eikenella, Kingella

- What are three medications often combined as a first line treatment for H. pylori?

    Omeprazole, clarithromycin and amoxicillin (PPI + 2 Antibioitcs)

- What is the prophylactic antibiotic most commonly given before a dental procedure if one is necessary?

    Amoxicillin 2 grams po 1 hour before procedure

- A pregnant woman and cat litter should make you think of what diagnosis?

    Toxoplasmosis

- What is the drug of choice to treat a urethritis caused by neisseria?

    Ceftriaxone (Rocephin)

- Is Klebsiella gram (+) or gram (-)?

    Gram (-)

- A Gram-positive organism in clusters should make you think of what diagnosis?

    Staph

- What is the best test for diagnosing Rocky Mountain spotted fever?

    Indirect immunofluorescent antibodies

- A Gram-negative coccobaccili found in the sputum of patient with pneumonia should make you think of what diagonsis?

    H. flu

- What medication is used as prophylaxis for meningococcal meningits?

    Rifampin

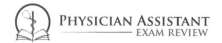

OB-GYN

- The secretory phase of the menstrual cycle (day 14-28) is dominated by what hormone? — *Progesterone*

- Is a nulliparous or mulitparous woman more likely to get preeclampsia? — *Nulliparity is a risk factor for preeclampsia.*

- Since a genetic cause is the number one reason for primary amenorrhea what is one very important test? — *Karyotype*

- Purulent cervical discharge should make you think of what diagnosis? — *Neisseria gonorrhoeae*

- A description of a young girl with a web neck or wide shield chest should make you think of what diagnosis? — *Turner's syndrome*

- A cervical biopsy comes back as CIN1. What is the next step? — *Repeat pap smear in 6 months and repeat colposcopy in 12 months.*

- What is the most common cause of secondary amenorrhea? — *Pregnancy*

- What three labs should you order if you are considering secondary amenorrhea? — *beta-HCG, TSH, Prolactin*

- Define premature birth. — *Delivery before 37 weeks.*

- A unilateral, single, mobile, firm, nontender solid breast mass should make you think of what diagnosis? — *Fibroadenoma*

- Define metrorrhagia. — *Bleeding between menstrual cycles.*

- Postmenopausal bleeding is immediately believed to be what diagnosis? — *Endometrial cancer until proven otherwise.*

OB-GYN

During what portion of the menstrual cycle does PMS occur?	*By definition it is in the second half and menstruation should relieve the symptoms.*
How do you treat bacterial vaginosis?	*Metronidazole x 7 days*
What location within the pelvis is endometriosis most commonly found?	*On an ovary*
What lab test is the gold standard for chlamydia?	*Nucleic acid amplification test*
Are fibrocystic breast masses usually bilateral or unilateral?	*Bilateral*
How do you definitively diagnose endometriosis?	*Exploratory laparoscopy*
What is the most common uterine tumor?	*Leiomyoma, also known as fibroids*
What ethnic background is at an increased risk of fibroids?	*African Americans are 5x more likely to have fibroids compared to Caucasian women.*
How do you treat vaginal candida?	*Fluconazole po 1 dose or azole cream x 1 week*
What is the first step of treatment for endometrial cancer?	*Total hysterectomy and bilateral salpingo-oophorectomy*
If you see the term chocolate cyst, it should make you think of what diagnosis?	*Endometrioma*
A surge in what hormone leads to ovulation?	*Luteinizing hormone (LH)*
A patient presents with irregular menses, hirsutism and infertility. What is the most likely diagnosis?	*Polycystic ovarian syndrome*
What endocrine issue is associated with PCOS?	*Insulin insensitivity*

OB-GYN

- You have a patient with PCOS who would like to get pregnant. What are two medications you may start her on?

    Metformin and Clomid

- What is the medical treatment for an early ectopic pregnancy?

    Methotrexate

- An ovarian cyst that contains hair and teeth should make you think of what diagnosis?

    Teratoma

- What is the mean age for ovarian cancer?

    63, you will need to think of this in an older patient with vague abdominal symptoms.

- Define the second stage of labor.

    Fully dilated to delivery

- A 66 year old female patient presents with bouts of nausea, weight loss and vague abdominal pain. What is the most likely diagnosis?

    Ovarian cancer

- When is it recommended to begin pap smears?

    Guidelines suggest beginning at age 21 regardless of sexual history.

- A cervical biopsy comes back as CIN2 or CIN3. What is your next step?

    Excision - LEEP, Cold knife (worry about incompetent cervix), Cryotherapy

- List two risk factors for cervical cancer.

    Multiple sexual partners, smoking

- How much time needs to pass before diagnosing secondary amenorrhea?

    If cycles have been normal 3 months. If cycles have been irregular 6 months.

- What is a cystocele?

    A herniation of the bladder into the vagina.

- What is the treatment for Turner's syndrome?

    Cyclical estrogen and progesterone

OB-GYN

What are three treatments for uterine prolapse?	*Pessary, Kegel's maneuvers, surgical repair*
What is the most common organism that causes mastitis?	*Staph aureus*
At approximately how many weeks pregnant is the uterus at the level of the umbilicus?	*20 weeks*
What is the most common cause of postpartum hemorrhage?	*Uterine atony*
Define missed abortion.	*No vaginal bleeding, cervix is closed, products of conception are still inside.*
At what age is primary amenorrhea diagnosed?	*Age 14 if no secondary sex characteristics. Age 16 if some secondary development.*
What is the first line treatment for mastitis?	*Dicloxacillin is first line. Cephalexin or erythromycin are second line.*
Should a breast feeding mother stop breast feeding if she develops mastitis?	*Mastitis is not a reason to stop breast feeding, but an abscess is.*
A physical exam revealing a retroverted uterus or uterosacral ligament nodularity should make you think of what diagnosis?	*Endometriosis*
At how many weeks of pregnancy can an amniocentesis be done?	*15-20 weeks*
List four risk factors for breast cancer?	*BRCA1 or BRCA2 positive, unopposed estrogen, nulliparity, early menarche, late menopause*
What is the average age of menopause?	*51*

OB-GYN

Cottage cheese discharge should make you think of what diagnosis?	*Vaginal candidiasis*
The follicular phase of menstruation is dominated by what hormone?	*Estrogen*
About how much weight should a woman gain during pregnancy?	*20-35 lbs*
Thin, sticky, malodorous vaginal discharge should make you think of what diagnosis?	*Bacterial vaginosis*
Vaginal infection with motile flagellated protozoa should make you think of what diagnosis?	*Trichomonas vaginitis*
List two medications commonly used for hypertension in pregnancy.	*Methyldopa and labetalol*
What is the classic triad of pre-eclampsia?	*HTN, edema and proteinuria*
Why is ovarian cancer so hard to diagnose?	*There are no good markers and the symptoms are very vague.*
What are two important things you need to tell you patients before putting them on metronidazole?	*Stay out of the sun and avoid alcohol.*
Define inevitable abortion.	*Vaginal bleeding, cervix is open, products of conception are still inside*
How is the first day of the menstrual cycle defined?	*The first day of menstrual bleeding is the first day of the cycle.*
What is the karyotype for a patient with Turner's syndrome?	*(45, X) They are missing one sex chromosome.*
Give the definition for preterm labor.	*Contractions that open the cervix before 37 weeks.*

OB-GYN

- A patient presents with mucopurulent discharge and cervical motion tenderness. What is the most likely diagnosis?

    Chlamydia - cervicitis

- Which four human papillomaviruses are linked to cervical cancer?

    HPV 16, 18, 31 and 33

- Clue cells should make you think of what diagnosis?

    Bacterial vaginosis

- What is the hallmark physical exam finding for placenta previa?

    Trick question - NEVER do a physical exam on someone with presumed placenta previa.

- What medium do you need to grow out Neisseria gonorrhoeae?

    Thayer-Martin

- What age range is the HPV vaccination recommended for?

    9 to 26 years old

- A patient with primary amenorrhea and a low FSH should make you think of what diagnosis?

    Hypothalamic pituitary insufficiency

- What characteristic of pelvic inflammatory disease will help to differentiate it in a question stem from ectopic pregnancy, appendicitis, ovarian torsion and ovarian cyst?

    It will be bilateral pain. Most other common abdominal complaints have unilateral pain.

- List 2 risk factors for ovarian cancer.

    BRCA1, family history, nulliparity, late menopause, Caucasian, Asian

- Define abortion.

    Delivery of uterine contents before 20 weeks.

- Does mastitis tend to be unilateral or bilateral?

    Unilateral and only one quadrant

- Define full term.

    Delivery at 37-42 weeks

OB-GYN

- When does quickening occur?

  Nulliparous 18-20 weeks, multiparous 14-16 weeks

- List three risk factors for placental abruption.

  HTN, smoking, AMA, cocaine use, PROM

- What is the treatment for ovarian cancer?

  Total hysterectomy and bilateral salpingo-oophorectomy. Then chemo and radiation.

- A patient believes she is pregnant. You notice that her cervix appears a little blue. What is the name of this sign?

  Chadwick's sign

- At approximately how many weeks pregnant is the uterus at the level of the symphysis pubis?

  12 weeks

- A snowstorm appearance on ultrasound should make you think of what diagnosis?

  Hydatidiform mole

- What medication can be used to control bleeding due to uterine atony?

  Oxytocin (Pitocin)

- What is the term for when the placenta has implanted directly over the cervical os?

  Placenta previa

- At how many weeks of pregnancy can chorionic villus sampling be done?

  10-13 weeks

- Why is folic acid given as a prenatal vitamin?

  Low folic acid can lead to neural tube defects.

- What is the most common endometrial cancer?

  75% are adenocarcinomas

- A strawberry cervix with copious yellow/green discharge should make you think of what diagnosis?

  Trichomonas vaginitis

OB-GYN

What organism causes us to warn pregnant patients to stay away from deli meats and soft cheeses?	Listeria
The baby was delivered several minutes ago. Suddenly there is a increase in blood flow from the vagina and the cord noticeably lengthens. What is the most likely cause of these signs?	Placental separation
What are two medications used to induce labor?	Cervidil (Prostoglandin gel applied to the cervix) which encourages cervical rippening and oxytocin which encourages uterine contractions.
As part of the antepartum testing a baby has a positive stress test. What does that mean?	They have had two heart rate accelerations in a 20 minute period of 15 beats above baseline for at least 15 seconds. This is a good thing.
Is FSH high or low in Turner's syndrome?	High, there are no ovaries to respond to FSH and so there is no negative feedback.
What is the most common type of ovarian cyst?	Functional cyst - no treatment necessary.
Define threatened abortion.	Vaginal bleeding, closed cervix, products of conception are still inside
List 4 risk factors for endometrial cancer.	Chronic unopposed estrogen, nulliparity, early menarche, late menopause, tamoxifen, DM, obesity, HTN, breast CA, ovarian CA
What would you expect to see on a KOH prep if the patient had vaginal candidiasis?	Pseudohyphae

OB-GYN

What is the #1 cause of septic arthritis in sexually active young adults?	*Neisseria gonorrhoeae*
How many days after conception is a serum beta-HCG positive?	*8*
If the pap smear results come back anything other than negative or ASCUS what is your next step?	*Colposcopy and biopsy*
List three risk factors for an ectopic pregnancy.	*Previous ectopic, scarred tubes (hx of PID or salpingitis), IUD*
Grape-like vesicles or a sack of grapes on ultrasound should make you think of what diagnosis?	*Hydatidiform mole*
What medication is used to increase surfactant levels and help with lung maturity if you are worried about preterm labor?	*Betamethasone*
What are two tocolytic medications you should be aware of?	*Magnesium sulfate and calcium channel blockers*
A woman presents to the ER concerned she is in preterm labor. What treatment should you begin before even getting any imaging or lab results?	*Give IV fluids (most often the patient is suffereing from dehydration).*
The pap smear results on a 23 year old patient come back as atypical squamous cell uncertain significance (ASCUS). What is your next step?	*Repeat pap smear in 12 months although HPV test is acceptable.*
What are three ways you can check for ruptured membranes?	*Ferning pattern on a slide, visualize leakage from the cervix, pooling in the vagina*
What is the normal range of fetal heart rate?	*120-160*

OB-GYN

Define menorrhagia.	Heavy prolonged menstrual flow
What Rh combination for mom and dad might cause the mother to create antiboides against the baby's red blood cells?	Mom Rh-negative and dad Rh-positive
At what point during pregnancy is RhoGAM given if it is needed?	28 weeks
Define complete abortion.	Vaginal bleeding, cervix open, products of conception have passed
Gestational diabetes puts mom and baby at increased risk of for what three things?	Preeclampsia, macrosomia (traumatic birth), slowing in fetal lung development
Which is associated with painful third trimester bleeding placental abruption or placenta previa?	Placental abruption
What are three causes for a postpartum hemorrhage?	Uterine atony, genital laceration, retained placenta
Define the third stage of labor.	Delivery of baby to delivery of placenta
What medication(s) are used to treat a postpartum metritis?	Clindamycin and gentamicin together
What is the most common sexually transmitted bacteria?	Chlamydia
Interference with work or school is part of which diagnosis, premenstrual syndrome or premenstrual dysphoric disorder?	Premenstrual dysphoric disorder
Which reproductive cancer carries the highest rates of death in women?	Ovarian cancer

OB-GYN

What is the most common infection following a C-section?	Metritis
How do you treat a Trichomonas infection?	Metronidazole
Define incomplete abortion.	Vaginal bleeding, cervix is open, products of conception partially passed
What is the most common site of an ectopic pregnancy?	Within a fallopian tube
Early on in pregnancy serial beta-HCG should double over what time period?	every 48-72 hours
Define procidentia.	Uterine prolapse beyond the introitus
What is the more popular term for Stein-Leventhal syndrome?	Polycystic ovarian syndrome
What is the formula for calculating estimated date of confinement or due date?	First day of last menstrual period + 7 days - 3 months
What are the five components of the biophysical profile as part of antepartum testing?	A non-stress test, fetal breathing, two gross body movements, fetal tone, amniotic fluid index
Define the first stage of labor.	Onset of contractions to full dilation of the cervix.
A rope-like breast mass should make you think of what diagnosis?	Fibrocystic breast mass

OPHTHAMOLOGY

What should a primary care provider do for a presumed retinal detachment?	Refer & position patient with head down
In what age range do you expect to most commonly find amaurosis fugax?	Patients older than 50
What is the #1 cause of retinal artery occlusion?	Carotid atherosclerotic disease.
When treating herpes keratitis should you use topical antivirals, topical steroids or both?	Don't use steroids. Topical antiviral and refer!
A patient describes his vision loss as a curtain coming down and then going back up. What might the diagnosis be?	Amaurosis fugax
A patient presents with a painful, red nodule on the eyelid. What diagnosis should you be thinking of? What treatment should you begin with?	Hordeolum (sty). Warm compress and progress to topical antibiotics if necessary.
A fundal exam shows a cherry-red spot. What diagnosis should you be thinking of?	Central retinal artery occlusion
A college student presents with a little purulent drainage from one eye and nontender preauricular lymphadenopathy. What diagnosis and pathogen should you be thinking of?	Chlamydia conjunctivitis
What should a primary care provider do for presumed central retinal artery occlusion?	Ophthalmic emergency! Refer and intermittent pressure and release of the eye.
A patient presents with unilateral blurriness developing over a few days. Fundal exam shows a "blood and thunder" pattern. What is the most likely diagnosis?	Central vein occlusion
What is appropriate treatment for central vein occlusion?	Typically self limited. Treat underlying disease.

OPHTHAMOLOGY

Is glaucoma more prevalent in males or females?	Females 3:1
Give two risk factors for glaucoma.	African American descent and diabetes
What is the yellow, brown fleshy mass on the conjunctiva which usually does not interfere with vision?	Pinguecula
A fundal exam shows a cup to disc ratio of >0.5. There are also vessels bending over the disc. What is the most likely diagnosis?	Glaucoma
A patient presents saying that he doesn't seem to need his glasses anymore after 30 yrs. What is the most likely diagnosis?	Cataract
A patient has metamorphopsia and a central blind spot. What is the most likely diagnosis?	Macular degeneration
What is the most likely quadrant for a retinal detachment?	Superior temporal
A patient presents with pain in one eye. The cornea is hazy and the pupils are fixed. What is the most likely diagnosis?	Glaucoma
What is the most common way of testing for metamorphopsia?	Amsler grid
You notice drusen deposits on fundal exam. What is the most likely diagnosis?	Macular degeneration
A patient presents with irritated, burning and tearing eyes. You notice some scurf and scales. Where do you begin treatment?	This is blepharitis. Treatment begins with good hygiene and moves on to topical antibiotics if necessary.

OPHTHAMOLOGY

☐	A patient has a history of multiple stys. He now has a painless nodule on his eyelid and minor conjunctivitis. What is the most likely diagnosis?	*Chalazion*
☐	What are the most common colors lost in color blindness?	*Red and green*
☐	What is the term for eyelids that turn in?	*Entropion*
☐	What is the term for bilateral yellow plaques near the eyes?	*Xanthelasma*
☐	A fundal exam shows an opalescent retina and boxcarring of arterioles. What is the most likely diagnosis?	*Central retinal artery occlusion*
☐	What is the most common preceding event for orbital cellulitis?	*URI*
☐	Vision loss described as curtain coming down should make you think of what diagnosis?	*Retinal detachment*
☐	You notice a bowing of the iris on exam. What is the most likely diagnosis?	*Glaucoma*
☐	A CT scan of the head shows broad infiltration of orbital fat. What is the most likely diagnosis?	*Orbital cellulitis*
☐	A patient presents with watery bilateral discharge from the eyes and nontender preauricular adenopathy. What is the most likely diagnosis? What is the most common pathogen?	*Viral conjunctivitis, adenovirus*
☐	How do you test for color blindness?	*Ishihara plates*
☐	A patient with a history of asthma presents complaining of stringy discharge from both eyes and severe swelling around the eyes. What is the most likely diagnosis?	*Allergic conjunctivitis*

OPHTHAMOLOGY

- What is the name for the triangular or wedge shaped growth on the conjunctiva that may interfere with vision?

    Pterygium

- What is the name of the test for dry eyes?

    Schirmer's test

- A patient having recently undergone cataract surgery presents complaining of vision loss in the operative eye. What is the most likely diagnosis?

    Retinal detachment

- A patient presents with sudden painless complete unilateral vision loss. What is the most likely diagnosis?

    Central retinal artery occlusion

- A dendritic lesion is seen with fluorescein stain. What is the most likely diagnosis?

    Herpes keratitis

- Which nerve is involved in herpes zoster ophthalmicus?

    Trigeminal nerve, CN 5

- Your attending asks you to come and see an excellent example of Hutchinson's sign. What diagnosis does the patient have?

    Herpes zoster ophthalmicus

- A patient presents with a dense corneal infiltrate and an epithelial defect seen with fluorescein stain. What diagnosis should you be thinking of?

    Corneal ulcer

- A feathery border in an eye exam should make you think of what diagnosis?

    Fungal infection

- A patient in the recovery room following foot surgery is complaining of severe photophobia. She feels as though there is something in her eye. What is the most likely diagnosis?

    Corneal abrasion (pt's scratch their eyes before they are completely awake from anesthesia)

- What is the treatment for subconjunctival hemorrhage?

    Reassurance

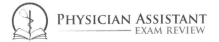

OPHTHAMOLOGY

☐ A 19 year old male took an elbow to the face while playing basketball this morning. The whole left side of his face is swollen and he can't look up. What is the most likely diagnosis?	*Orbital fracture*
☐ A patient complains of seeing halos and rainbows around lights. She also complains of moderate photophobia? What is the most likely diagnosis?	*Glaucoma*
☐ What is the first thing you should be thinking of if a pediatric patient comes in with blood in the anterior chamber of the eye (hyphema).	*Child abuse until proven otherwise*
☐ How long after a radiant energy burn do symptoms typically show?	*6-12 hours*
☐ What is the term for eyelids that turn out?	*Ectropion*
☐ What is the initial treatment for a chemical burn to the eyes?	*Irrigate, irrigate, irrigate*
☐ Color blindness is transmitted through what genetic pattern?	*Dominant X-linked*
☐ What is the term for being nearsighted? What type of lens do you use to correct it?	*Myopia, concave lenses*
☐ A college student presents with copious purulent drainage from one eye. What is the most likely diagnosis?	*Neisseria conjunctivitis*
☐ What is the first line treatment for orbital cellulitis?	*IV antibiotics, followed by 2 weeks of oral antibiotics*
☐ What is the term for being farsighted? What type of lens do you use to correct it?	*Hyperopia, convex*
☐ What is tonometry used for?	*Determining intraocular pressure*

PULMONOLOGY

What is the most common patient complaint with emphysema?	Shortness of breath
At what age should vaccinations for pneumococcal pneumonia begin?	65 years old
Prolonged expiration (low FEV1) should make you think of what diagnosis?	Asthma or COPD
Hampton's hump on CXR should make you think of what diagnosis?	Pulmonary embolism
How long after administering a PPD should it be read?	48-72 hours
A patient without a functioning spleen is more susceptible to what type of organisms?	Encapsulated organisms most commonly Strep pneumoniae and H. Flu.
What is the most common cause of pneumonia in children less than 1 year old?	Respiratory syncytial virus (RSV)
What is the treatment for pneumocystis jiroveci pneumonia?	Bactrim
What occupations are associated with berylliosis?	Aerospace and nuclear plant workers
What CXR finding might make you think of berylliosis?	Diffuse infiltrates with hilar adenopathy
What is the gold standard for diagnosis of a pleural effusion?	Thoracocentesis
When performing a decompression for a tension pneumothorax where do you put the needle?	2nd intercostal space at the midclavicular line
Oseltamivir (Tamiflu) may be given to children above what age?	1 year old

PULMONOLOGY

☐	Zanamivir (Relenza) may be give to children above what age?	*7 years old*
☐	An HIV patient with ground glass appearance on CXR should make you think of what diagnosis?	*Pneumocystis jiroveci pneumonia (PJP used to be know as PCP)*
☐	A noncaseating granuloma should make you think of what diagnosis?	*Sarcoidosis*
☐	A pearl formation on CXR should make you think of what diagnosis?	*Squamous cell lung cancer*
☐	Ghon or Ranke complexes on CXR should make you think of what diagnosis?	*TB*
☐	A Westermark sign on CXR should make you think of what diagnosis?	*Pulmonary embolism*
☐	Mesothelioma is most commonly found in what lung location?	*80% are found in the pleural lining*
☐	What CXR finding might make you think of mesothelioma?	*Pleural thickening, remember 80% are found in the pleura lining*
☐	Hyperinflation on a CXR as well as eosinophilia on CBC should make you think of what diagnosis?	*Asthma*
☐	What organism is the most common cause of pneumonia in a patient with cystic fibrosis?	*Pseudomonas*
☐	A college student presents with pneumonia. What two organisms should you be thinking of?	*Chlamydia and mycoplasma*
☐	At what size induration would a PPD be positive for an HIV patient?	*5mm*

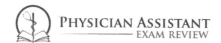

PULMONOLOGY

- You suspect a pneumothorax. What instructions should go along with the order for a CXR?

    It should be an end expiratory view in order to look for visceral pleural air.

- List the three most commonly used medical treatments for COPD?

    Oxygen, ipratropium and albuterol

- List 4 medications which may cause asthma.

    Beta blockers, NSAIDS, ACEI, ASA

- Nodular opacities in the upper lung fields should make you think of what diagnosis?

    Silicosis

- What is the initial treatment for active TB?

    INH+RIF+PZA+EMB x several months typically followed by INH+RIF once sensativities come back

- Caseating granulomas should make you think of what diagnosis?

    TB

- Blue bloater refers to the characteristic physical exam findings of what disease?

    Chronic bronchitis

- A contralateral mediastinal shift should make you think of what diagnosis?

    Tension pneumothorax

- What is the best test to diagnose bronchiectasis?

    CT

- What are the main side effects of isoniazid?

    Hepatitis and peripheral neuropathy

- You are treating a patient for TB. He has noticed that his body fluids now have an orange tint. What drug is most likely causing this?

    Rifampin

- Ethambutol has what two major side effects?

    Optic neuritis, red green vision loss

- If you see a question with anything to do with rats and the patient has pneumonia, what organism should you be thinking of?

    Yersinia pestis

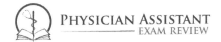

PULMONOLOGY

- What is the most common organism causing pneumonia in COPD patients? — *Haemophilus influenzae*

- Where is a Pancoast tumor found on CXR? — *At the apex of either the right or left lung*

- Will evidence of TB be seen more frequently in the upper or lower lung lobes on CXR? — *Upper*

- A patient has pneumonia with rust colored sputum. What is the most likely diagnosis? — *Strep pneumonia*

- Coal miners lung often shows nodular opacities in what lung fields? — *Upper lung fields*

- When you step up the diagnosis from intermittent asthma to mild persistent asthma what medication should you add? — *An inhaled steroid like fluticasone*

- Any question about rabbits and pneumonia should make you think of what diagnosis? — *Tularemia*

- Dullness to percussion should make you think of what diagonsis? — *Lobar pneumonia*

- A young child presents to ER and you see him waiting in tripod position. What is the most likely diagnosis? — *Epiglottitis*

- At what size induration would a PPD be positive for a healthcare worker? — *10mm*

- List six extrapulmonary complications of lung cancer. — *SPHERE - SVC syndrome, Pancoast tumor, Horner's syndrome, Endocrine problems, Recurrent laryngeal symptoms, Effusions (exudative)*

- Currant jelly sputum should make you think of what diagnosis? — *Klebsiella pneumoniae*

PULMONOLOGY

What happens to total lung capacity in sarcoidosis?	It goes down
What will the likely findings be on a CXR of a patient with asbestosis?	Linear opacities at the bases with pleural plaques
Tympany to percussion should make you think of what diagonsis?	Large pneuomthorax
What are the three most common cancers to metastasize to the lungs?	Breast, liver and colon
A thumbprint sign on x-ray should make you think of what two diagnoses?	Lateral C-spine = epiglottitis, abdominal = intestinal ischemia
A barrel chest should make you think of what diagnosis?	Emphysema
Are the lungs noisy or quiet in COPD?	Quiet
List four indications for the flu vaccine.	Child 6-59 months, pregnant female, healthcare worker, age greater than 50
Posttussive rales should make you think of what diagnosis?	TB
Bullae and blebs on CXR should make you think of what diagnosis?	Emphysema
Rhonci or wheezes that clear after coughing suggest what diagnosis?	Bronchitis or atelectasis
Does FEV1 go up or down with asthma?	It goes down
A very sick patient with diffuse infiltrates that spare the costophrenic angles should make you think of what diagnosis?	Acute respiratory distress syndrome (ARDS)
What is the most common cause of bronchiectasis?	Cystic Fibrosis

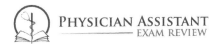

PULMONOLOGY

What is the gold standard for the diagnosis of cystic fibrosis?	Sweat chloride test
An exudative pleural effusion should make you think of what diagnosis?	TB, Lung cancer
What is the treatment for epiglottitis?	2nd or 3rd generation cephalosporin (ceftriaxone), macrolides may also be used (clindamycin)
Transudative pleural effusions should make you think of what diagnosis?	Congestive heart failure
What two lung cancers are typically found centrally on CXR?	Small cell and squamous cell
What two lung cancers are typically found peripherally on CXR?	Adenocarcinoma and Large cell
Pertussis is most commonly treated with what antibiotic?	Erythromycin
List the four most common places lung cancer will metastasize to.	Bone, brain, adrenals and liver
If you come across a question where the patient has erythema nodosum and an enlarged parotid gland what is the most likely diagnosis?	Sarcoidosis
What is erythema nodosum?	Tender red nodules usually found on the shins.
A thin looking heart and flattened diaphragm on CXR should make you think of what diagnosis?	Emphysema
If you see a question with an alcoholic who has been diagnosed with pneumonia what is the most likely organism?	Klebsiella pneumoniae

PULMONOLOGY

Honeycombing and tram tracks on the CXR should make you think of what diagnosis?	Bronchiectasis and idopathic pulmonary fibrosis
Paradoxical pulses may be found in what pulmonary disorder?	Asthma
An older patient presents with pneumonia and diarrhea. What is the most likely diagnosis?	Legionella pneumonia
Eggshell opacities on the CXR should make you think of what diagnosis?	Silicosis
List three causes of decreased tactile fremitus.	COPD, asthma, pleural effusion, pneumothorax
Hyperresonance to percussion should make you think of what diagnosis?	Emphysema, pneumothorax, asthma
If you hear crackles in the lung fields list three pulmonary issues that should be in your differential.	Pneumonia, fibrosis, CHF, Bronchitis
Does total lung capacity go up or down in COPD?	It goes up.
List three things that should be in your differential if you hear wheezes on a lung exam?	Asthma, COPD, Bronchitis
What is it called when a patient says "ee" but on auscultion you here "ay"?	Egophony
A physical exam finding of egophony should make you think of what diagonsis?	Lobar pneumonia
A CXR shows vascular redistribution and blurred vascular outlines. What is the most likely diagnosis?	CHF

GASTROINTESTINAL

- What is the term for difficulty swallowing?

    Dysphagia

- Bird-beak esophagus on barium swallow should make you think of what diagnosis?

    Achalasia

- What is the most common location for an anal fissure?

    Posterior midline

- Crohn's is found where in the GI tract?

    It can be from esophagus to anus.

- What does HBsAg (hep B surface antigen) indicate?

    Active Hep B infection

- How do you treat achalasia?

    Loosen up the muscle - botox, dilation or surgery

- A corkscrew appearance on barium study should make you think of what diagnosis?

    Esophageal spasms

- Epigastric abdominal pain which radiates to the back should make you think of what diagnosis?

    Pancreatitis

- In order to contract hepatitis D what must you already have?

    Hepatitis B

- Left lower quadrant pain and tenderness should make you think of what diagnosis?

    Diverticulitis

- What is the treatment for most Mallory-Weiss tears?

    Watchful waiting, these will typically resolve within 48 hours.

- A thumbprint sign on an abdominal film should make you think of what diagnosis?

    Intestinal ischemia

- What will the bowel sounds be early on in a small bowel obstruction? What will they be later on?

    Early they are hyperactive. Late they are absent.

GASTROINTESTINAL

- A patient has had GERD for years. Over the past year, he has noticed an increase in difficulty swallowing his food. This should make you think of what diagnosis?

    Esophageal strictures

- What are two treatments you should consider for esophageal strictures?

    Dilation of the esophagus and long term PPIs.

- What are two common predisposing factors for esophageal varices?

    Portal HTN and cirrhosis often caused by alcoholism.

- What is a common symptom that goes along with chest pain for GERD patients?

    Dry cough

- What medication is most commonly used for long term treatment of GERD?

    Proton pump inhibitors - omeprazole, lansoprazole, pantoprazole

- What is the imaging modality of choice for pancreatitis?

    CT

- What is the best test to check for H. pylori?

    Urea breath test

- Is peptic ulcer disease more common in the duodenum or the stomach?

    Duodenum

- What is the most common location for a pancreatic tumor?

    75% occur in the head of the pancreas.

- With a gastric ulcer are the patient's symptoms exacerbated or relieved with food?

    Exacerbated

- Fasting gastrin will be above what level with gastrinoma?

    >150 pg/ml

- Projectile vomiting should make you think of what diagnosis?

    Pyloric stenosis

- Most gallstones are made of what substance?

    Cholesterol

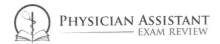

GASTROINTESTINAL

☐	What is the name of the sign when a patient shows inhibited inspiration with pressure over the RUQ? What diagnosis does it suggest?	Murphy's sign, Cholecystitis
☐	What is the most specific test for acute cholecystitis?	HIDA
☐	What is the gold standard for diagnosis and treatment of bile duct stones?	ERCP
☐	What is Charcot's triad?	RUQ pain, fever, jaundice
☐	What is Reynold's pentad and why does it matter?	Charcot's triad + hypotension + altered mental status. It indicates high risk of sepsis.
☐	What disease is defined as an immunologic response to gluten?	Celiac
☐	What is the main risk factor for esophagitis?	Immunocompromised patient
☐	An endoscopy for presumed esophagitis shows multiple shallow ulcers. What is the most likely diagnosis?	Herpes simplex virus
☐	List two common offending agents for pill induced esophagitis?	NSAIDS, KCl, iron, antibiotics
☐	A 30 year old African American woman presents with dysphagia. You notice she also has thickened skin. A barium swallow demonstrates the absence of peristalsis. What is the most likely diagnosis?	Scleroderma
☐	A patient complains of regurgitating undigested food several hours after a meal. What is the most likely diagnosis?	Zenker's diverticulum
☐	What is the most common cause of peptic ulcer disease?	H. pylori

GASTROINTESTINAL

What is the most specific diagnostic test for peptic ulcer disease?	*Endoscopy*
What is the only curative therapy for gastric adenocarcinoma?	*Surgical resection*
A patient presents complaining of right upper quadrant pain 20 minutes after meals. What is the most likely diagnosis?	*Cholecystitis*
What does ERCP stand for?	*Endoscopic retrograde cholangiopancreatography*
What is the most common cause of acute bacterial cholangitis?	*Choledocholithiasis*
Onion ring fibrosis from a bile duct biopsy should make you think of what diagnosis?	*Primary sclerosing cholangitis*
What two viral hepatitis infections are self limiting?	*Hepatitis A and hepatitis E*
Pica is often related to what type of anemia?	*Iron deficiency anemia*
What does an Anti-HBc (hep B core antibody) indicate?	*Previous or ongoing hepatitis B infection*
What does Anti-HBs (hep B surface antibody) indicate?	*Recovery from infection or immunization to hepatitis B*
What it is the recommended treatment for hepatitis C infection?	*Pegylated interferon alpha-2*
What medication used in hepatitis B infection helps prevent the need for liver transplant?	*Lamivudine*
There are vaccines for which two versions of hepatitis?	*Hepatitis A and hepatitis B*

GASTROINTESTINAL

- Will a patient with achalasia have dysphagia to liquids, solids or both?

    Both

- If you have heartburn that does not improve with medication what is the most likely diagnosis?

    Gastrinoma

- What are the two main complications of cirrhosis?

    Portal HTN & liver insufficiency

- What is a good beta blocker to reduce portal HTN?

    Propranolol

- What tumor marker may be used for liver cancer?

    alpha-Fetoprotein

- What are the two most common causes of pancreatitis?

    Cholelithiasis and ETOH

- Describe Cullen's sign.

    Umbilical ecchymosis often related to pancreatitis.

- What are the 5 points of Ranson's criteria on admission?

    older than 55, WBC>16, glucose>200, LDH>350, AST>250

- What is the first step in treating GERD?

    Lifestyle modification

- Steatorrhea should make you think of what diagnosis?

    Pancreatitis

- Describe Courvoisier's sign.

    Nontender, palpable gallbladder which may indicate pancreatic neoplasm.

- What tumor marker can be used to follow pancreatic cancer?

    CA-19-9

- A patient complains of periumbilical pain which has now moved over McBurney's point. What is the most likely diagnosis?

    Appendicitis

GASTROINTESTINAL

Describe how to perform the psoas sign.	The patient is supine and attempts to raise the right leg against resistance.
What is the term for painful swallowing?	Odynophagia
Describe how to perform the obturator sign.	The patient is supine and attempts to flex and internally rotate right hip.
What is the best imaging study for acute appendicitis?	CT
What two blood test can be used to diagnose celiac?	IgA endomysial antibody and IgA tTG antibody
How much fiber should you normally get in a day?	About 30 grams
What treatment should be started for asymptomatic diverticulosis?	None
Is surgery curative for Crohn's or ulcerative colitis?	Ulcerative colitis
What causes Mallory-Weiss tears?	Forced vomiting or retching (often involving alcohol)
A colonoscopy that shows cobblestone or skip lesions should make you think of what diagnosis?	Crohn's disease
What class of medication is first line to treat inflammatory bowel disease in the maintenance phase?	5-ASA products - sulfasalazine, mesalamine
Currant jelly stool should make you think of what diagnosis?	Intussusception
Severe abdominal pain 30 minutes after a meal should make you think of what diagnosis?	Intestinal ischemia
What is the most common cause of lower GI bleed?	Diverticulosis

GASTROINTESTINAL

☐	What is the most common location of colorectal cancer?	*Cecum about 38%*
☐	Colorectal cancer patients are almost all older than what age?	*90% of patients are older than 50.*
☐	An epigastric olive-shaped mass should make you think of what diagnosis?	*Pyloric stenosis*
☐	An elevated serum amylase and lipase should make you think of what diagnosis?	*Pancreatitis*
☐	Under routine circumstances when should patients begin getting screening colonoscopies?	*Age 50*
☐	What is the #1 cause of small bowel obstruction?	*Postoperative adhesions*
☐	Air fluid levels on abdominal x-ray should make you think of what diagnosis?	*Bowel obstruction*
☐	Which is more likely to pass into the scrotum, a direct or indirect hernia?	*Indirect*
☐	A string sign on barium swallow should make you think of what diagnosis?	*Pyloric stenosis*
☐	What is the first line of treatment for an anal fissure?	*Fluid and fiber*
☐	What are two things that an anal fissure off midline might suggest?	*Crohn's, syphilis, HIV, neoplasm*
☐	What medical treatment is given for a gastrinoma?	*Proton pump inhibitors*
☐	What is the term for an abscess in the sacrococcygeal cleft?	*Pilonidal disease*

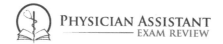

GASTROINTESTINAL

- How do you treat an H. pylori infection? — *PPI + 2 antibiotics, commonly omeprazole + clarithromycin and amoxicillin or PPI + metronidazole + tetracycline*

- Painless bright red blood per rectum should make you think of what diagnosis? — *Hemorrhoids*

- A patient on sulfasalazine for an inflammatory bowel disease should be supplemented with what vitamin? — *Folate*

- What is the most common anorectal problem affecting patients over 50? — *Hemorrhoids*

- A gastrinoma is also known as what syndrome? — *Zollinger-Ellison syndrome*

- Salivary amylase breaks down what macronutrient? — *Carbohydrates*

- What is the medical term for feeling like there is a lump in your throat? — *Globus*

- What is the most common vessel blocked with intestinal ischemia? — *Superior mesenteric artery*

- Describe Grey-Turner's sign. — *Flank ecchymosis often related to pancreatitis*

- What are the first three steps of managing pancreatitis? — *NPO, pain control, fluids*

- A patient presents with unproductive retching, acute localized epigastric distention and inability to pass a nasogastric tube. What is the most likely diagnosis? — *Gastric volvulus*

- What is the most common cause of a folate deficiency? — *Alcoholism*

GASTROINTESTINAL

☐ Should diverticulitis always be admitted?	*No, mild cases can be treated as outpatients with rest and clear fluids.*
☐ Which NSAID has the highest rate of peptic ulceration?	*Naproxen*
☐ What is the diagnostic test of choice for Zenker's diverticulum?	*Barium swallow will show the diverticulum.*
☐ What is the leading cause of iron deficiency anemia?	*Chronic GI bleed*
☐ At what age and how often should fecal occult blood tests be performed as a screening tool?	*Beginning at age 50, and they should be done every year.*
☐ How often should patients with pernicious anemia have a screening endoscopy performed?	*Every 5 years looking for signs of gastric carcinoma.*
☐ Are one half of all adult hernias direct or indirect inguinal hernias?	*Indirect inguinal hernias makeup 50% of all adult hernias.*
☐ How is celiac disease most commonly diagnosed?	*Endoscopic biopsy*
☐ Define pellagra?	*Niacin (B3) deficiency*
☐ An endoscopy for presumed esophagitis shows several solitary deep ulcers. What is the most likely diagnosis?	*Cytomegalovirus*
☐ Which are more painful, hemorrhoids above or below the dentate line?	*Below, internal hemorrhoids are not painful.*
☐ An abdominal exam with pain out of proportion to the exam should make you think of what diagnosis?	*Intestinal ischemia*
☐ Does adenocarcinoma arise from the proximal or distal esophagus?	*Distal*

PEDIATRICS

- German measles is also known as what disease?

    Rubella

- Bruises may be purple, green, yellow and brown. How many days old is a yellow bruise?

    Purple day 1-5, Green day 5-7, Yellow 7-10, Brown 10-14

- Pain with movement of the pinna or tragus should make you think of what diagnosis?

    Otitis externa

- What is the first line treatment for pertussis?

    Erythromycin

- By what age should a child be able to hold up her head?

    3 months

- A Salter-Harris type I fracture affects what area of the bone?

    Only the physis (growth plate).

- By what age should a child be able to sit up?

    6 months

- A 15 year old overweight boy presents to your office limping with knee pain. What is the most likely diagnosis?

    Slipped capital femoral epiphysis

- A premature infant with hyaline membrane disease will have what appearance on CXR?

    Bilateral atelectasis or ground glass appearance

- Atypical or walking pneumonia is caused by what pathogen?

    mycoplasma

- What antibiotic is the first line treatment for mycoplasma pneumonia?

    A macrolide, erythromycin or azithromycin

- A patient is having seizures along with a mouse-like odor from the urine. What diagnosis should you be thinking of?

    Phenylketonuria

- The description of a dew drop on a rose petal should make you think of what diagnosis?

    Chickenpox

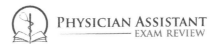

PEDIATRICS

Pale and boggy nasal mucosa should make you think of what diagnosis?	*Allergic rhinitis*
List the five major Jones criteria for diagnosing rheumatic fever.	*Polyarthritis, carditis, subcuticular nodes, erythema marginatum, chorea*
Describe erythema marginatum.	*Pink rings on the trunk and inner surfaces of the limbs.*
A child with bulky greasy stool should make you think of what diagnosis?	*Cystic fibrosis*
At what age should an infant begin cooing?	*2 months*
What is the most common cause of an upper respiratory tract infection?	*Rhinovirus*
Koplik spots are white clustered lesions on the buccal mucosa. What virus are they pathognomonic for?	*Measles/Rubeola*
What is the first line antibiotic for otitis media?	*Amoxicillin*
How do you treat a patient with respiratory syncytial virus?	*Albuterol, steroids and fluids*
A child presents with painful ulcers in his mouth. On physical exam you find more of the same type of ulcers on his feet and hands. What virus is most likely causing these symptoms?	*Coxsackie virus*
What is the gold standard for the diagnosis of cystic fibrosis?	*Sweat chloride test*
By what age should a child be able to walk?	*12 months*
If you believe there may be a foreign body obstructing a child's breathing what type of CXR should you order?	*Expiratory view looking for hyperinflation due to air trapping.*

PEDIATRICS

What is the medical term for lazy eye?	Amblyopia
A patient presents with a staccato cough but no fever. What is the most likely diagnosis?	Chlamydia pneumoniae
What is the most serious complication of Kawasaki syndrome?	Aortic Aneurysm
A musical vibratory murmur best heard at the apex in a child should make you think of what diagnosis?	Still's murmur
A palpable olive-shaped epigastric mass in a one month old should make you think of what diagnosis?	Pyloric stenosis
At what age should a child be able to use a spoon and stack 3-4 blocks?	18 months
What is the x-ray finding that supports diagnosis of a slipped capital femoral epiphysis?	Ice cream falling of the cone
Which viral exanthem often has conjunctivitis as one of it's symptoms?	Measles/Rubeola
What is the most common congenital heart defect?	Ventricular septal defect
A boot-shaped heart on CXR should make you think of what diagnosis?	Tetralogy of Fallot
During a physical exam of a child, you feel a tubular or sausage-shaped mass. What is the most likely diagnosis?	Intussusception
What is the treatment for a volvulus in a child?	Barium enema
By what age should a child be able to roll over?	4 months
What is pertussis more commonly referred to as?	Whooping cough

PEDIATRICS

Which heart valve is most associated with rheumatic fever?	*Mitral*
You hear a loud harsh holosystolic murmur in a child. It is heard best at the LLSB. What is the most likely diagnosis?	*Ventricular septal defect*
A child presents with paroxysmal abdominal pain, nausea, vomiting and diarrhea. What is the most likely diagnosis?	*Intussusception*
At what age should a child begin to feed himself?	*6 months*
Currant jelly stool should make you think of what diagnosis?	*Intussusception*
Is an upper respiratory infection which includes hoarseness most likely bacterial or viral?	*Viral*
Describe Barlow's test.	*Adduct and internal rotation of the hips*
A CXR finding of notched ribs in a child should make you think of what diagnosis?	*Coarctation of the aorta*
How long should you wait for a swallowed marble to pass through the body before considering surgery?	*24 hours*
A 4 year old boy presents between October and March with wheezing, coughing, a runny nose and increased respiratory rate. What is the most likely pathogen?	*Respiratory syncytial virus*
Describe the pattern of weight gain in an infant over the following time periods: week one, 6 months, 12 months, 3 years old and 4 years old.	*Newborns lose 10% of their birth weight initially but are back to birth weight at 10 days, 6m = 2x birth weight, 12m = 3x birthweight, 3 y/o= 30 lbs & 30 inches, 4 y/o = 40 lbs & 40 inches*

PEDIATRICS

By what age should a child be able to kick a ball?	*24 months*
A child with a fever lasting longer than five days should make you think of what diagnosis?	*Kawasaki syndrome*
A widely split fixed S2 should make you think of what diagnosis?	*Atrial septal defect*
Nasal polyps should make you think of what diagnosis?	*Cystic fibrosis*
In order to diagnose rheumatic fever what one thing must you have?	*Evidence of a strep infection either positive titer or positive culture. In addition to that you need 2 major criteria or 1 major and 2 minor criteria.*
Forchheimer spots are associated with what disease?	*Rubella*
A Salter-Harris type III fracture affects what area of the bone?	*The physis (growth plate) as well as the epiphysis*
A lacey pink rash on the face of a child should make you think of what diagnosis?	*Erythema infectiosum aka fifth disease aka slapped cheek*
Unilateral purulent rhinitis should make you think of what diagnosis?	*Foreign body*
What is the medical term for cross-eyed?	*Strabismus*
What organism is the most common cause of otitis media?	*Strep pneumonia*
At what age should a child begin to say momma and dadda?	*12 months*

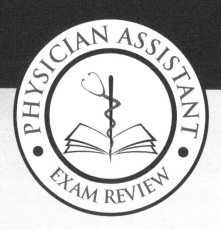

Section B is all 1200 questions From Section A in a completely random order. Here they are not grouped by topic. The questions are completely random. Start with the first page and move through from beginning to end. This section is best used in the couple of days leading up to your exam when you want to cover everything one last time. Good Luck!

B

What is the most common cause of sudden death?	Ventricular fibrillation
Color blindness is transmitted through what genetic pattern?	Dominant X-linked
A prostate biopsy consists of how many samples?	6 to 12
What is the definitive treatment for a patient with recurrent ventricular tachycardia?	Implanted defibrillator
How does ezetimibe work?	Decreases intestinal absorption of cholesterol
What is the drug of choice to treat C. difficile?	Metronidazole (Flagyl)
A patient on sulfasalazine for an inflammatory bowel disease should be supplemented with what vitamin?	Folate
A child presenting with an erythematous sandpaper rash should make you think of what diagnosis?	Scarlet fever
Owl eye inclusion bodies should make you think of what diagnosis?	Cytomegalovirus (CMV)
In a patient with aortic stenosis, will the PMI be medially displaced, normal or laterally displaced?	It will be laterally displaced due to left ventricular hypertrophy.
List two causes of right atrial enlargement.	Pulmonary HTN, severe lung disease, pulmonary valve stenosis
Acute endocarditis is most commonly caused by what organism?	Staph aureus
Describe erythema marginatum.	Pink rings on the trunk and inner surfaces of the limbs.

B

☐ A patient was camping a few days ago and now has a rash that began on his wrists and ankles. What diagnosis should you be thinking of?	*Rocky Mountain spotted fever*
☐ Clicking or locking of the knee indicates what diagnosis?	*Meniscal tear*
☐ Decreased GABA and substance P should make you think of what diagnosis?	*Huntington's*
☐ In order to contract hepatitis D what must you already have?	*Hepatitis B*
☐ How long does a panic attack typically last?	*10-20 minutes*
☐ What is the most common precipitating event for posttraumatic stress disorder in women?	*Rape*
☐ What is the best patient position to hear aortic regurge and aortic stenosis?	*Sitting up and leaning forward*
☐ An india ink stain showing cysts should make you think of what diagnosis?	*Cryptococcosis*
☐ At what point during pregnancy is RhoGAM given if it is needed?	*28 weeks*
☐ A 35 year old patient comes to your office because his wife made him. He has been increasingly irritable and moody. She has also noticed that he is very restless. You order a CT scan which shows cerebral atrophy as well as atrophy of the caudate nucleus. What diagnosis should you be thinking of?	*Huntington's disease*
☐ What is the accessory pathway associated with Wolff-Parkinson-White syndrome?	*The bundle of Kent*

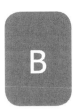

Ghon or Ranke complexes on CXR should make you think of what diagnosis?	TB
What does koilonychia refer to?	Spoon-shaped nails which may be found in microcytic anemia.
What is the therapeutic range for INR following an organic valve replacement?	2 to 3
A 35 year old female presents with heat intolerance, weight loss and palpitations. What diagnosis should you be thinking of?	Hyperthyroidism
What side effect might make a patient stop taking an ACEI?	Cough
What is the gold standard for the diagnosis of cystic fibrosis?	Sweat chloride test
Name two fibric acid derivatives.	Fenofibrate and gemfibrozil
Is sickle cell microcytic, macrocytic or normocytic?	Microcytic
A patient's wife complains that he is hypervigilant and has a hyperstartle response. What diagnosis should you be thinking of?	Posttraumatic stress disorder
A boot-shaped heart on CXR should make you think of what diagnosis?	Tetralogy of Fallot
What molecule binds iron in the blood stream?	Transferrin
What is a first line treatment for rheumatoid arthritis?	Methotrexate
Gestational diabetes puts mom and baby at increased risk of for what three things?	Preeclampsia, macrosomia (traumatic birth), slowing in fetal lung development

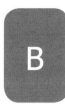

☐	What type of organism causes tetanus?	*A Gram + rod, Clostridium tetani*
☐	What drug do you use to treat pinworm?	*You treat everyone in the house with albendazole. Two weeks later you treat them again.*
☐	A physical exam revealing a retroverted uterus or uterosacral ligament nodularity should make you think of what diagnosis?	*Endometriosis*
☐	There is a sunburst appearance on x-ray. What is the most likely diagnosis?	*Osteosarcoma*
☐	How much more potent is T3 than T4?	*3-4x*
☐	What should a primary care provider do for a presumed retinal detachment?	*Refer & position patient with head down*
☐	Anti-Jo-1 antibodies should make you think of what diagnosis?	*Polymyositis*
☐	Is pseudomonas gram (+) or gram (−)?	*Gram (−)*
☐	A CXR finding of notched ribs in a child should make you think of what diagnosis?	*Coarctation of the aorta*
☐	A patient's lab work shows positive Smith antibody and positive double-stranded DNA antibodies. What is the most likely diagnosis?	*Lupus*
☐	What is the #1 cause of retinal artery occlusion?	*Carotid atherosclerotic disease*
☐	What is the most common cause of C-spine fractures?	*Motor vehicle accidents*
☐	Which herpesvirus causes Epstein–Barr?	*Herpes 4*
☐	What is the term for eyelids that turn in?	*Entropion*

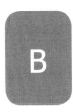

If you see the term chocolate cyst, it should make you think of what diagnosis?	Endometrioma
What fracture is the #1 cause of compartment syndrome?	Tibial shaft fracture
Define full term.	Delivery at 37-42 weeks
Nasal polyps should make you think of what diagnosis?	Cystic fibrosis
List four disease states in which you may find basophilic stippling.	Lead poisoning, beta or alpha thalassemia, sideroblastic anemia, arsenic poisoning
Is neisseria gram (+) or gram (-)?	Gram (-)
Coin-shaped plaques should make you think of what diagnosis?	Nummular eczema
Define metrorrhagia.	Bleeding between menstrual cycles.
A patient without a functioning spleen is more susceptible to what type of organisms?	Encapsulated organisms most commonly Strep pneumoniae and H. Flu.
A patient presents with irritated, burning and tearing eyes. You notice some scurf and scales. Where do you begin treatment?	This is blepharitis. Treatment begins with good hygiene and moves on to topical antibiotics if necessary.
What is the definitive treatment for atrial flutter?	Radiofrequency catheter ablation
Describe Grey-Turner's sign.	Flank ecchymosis often related to pancreatitis.
What is the only curative therapy for gastric adenocarcinoma?	Surgical resection

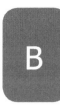

☐ What medication class is used to lower triglycerides?	*Fibric acid derivatives*
☐ Why can't you give fluoroquinolones to kids?	*They can cause cartilage development problems.*
☐ A patient has a tremor with motion in his hands. What medication might you prescribe?	*This patient has an active tremor therefore a beta blocker like propranolol is a good start.*
☐ A patient presents to your office complaining of a tremor in his right hand. He states after a beer it goes away completely. What diagnosis should you be thinking of?	*Benign essential tremor or familial tremor*
☐ What is the most common fracture in a patient with osteoporosis?	*A compression fracture of a vertebral body followed by hip fractures*
☐ What are three ways you can check for ruptured membranes?	*Ferning pattern on a slide, visualize leakage from the cervix, pooling in the vagina*
☐ What lab result will increase the risk of digoxin toxicity?	*Hypokalemia or hypercalcemia*
☐ Subacute endocarditis is most commonly caused by what organism?	*Strep Viridans*
☐ A patient presents with a staccato cough but no fever. What diagnosis should you be thinking of?	*Chlamydia pneumoniae*
☐ Cottage cheese discharge should make you think of what diagnosis?	*Vaginal candidiasis*
☐ An 82 year old patient complains of headaches and jaw claudication. What is the most likely diagnosis?	*Giant cell (temporal) arteritis*

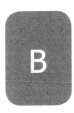

Eggshell opacities on the CXR should make you think of what diagnosis?	Silicosis and coal workers lung
What cranial nerve is affected with Bell's palsy?	CN VII
A middle age male presents with unilateral periorbital headaches occurring daily for several weeks. These headaches are extremely painful. Which type of headache is the most likely cause?	Cluster headache
A Gram-positive organism in clusters should make you think of what diagnosis?	Staph
What is tonometry used for?	Determining intraocular pressure
What two main causes should you be thinking of in a macrocytic anemia?	Malnutrition and severe blood loss
A patient presents with sudden painless complete unilateral vision loss. What diagnosis should you be thinking of?	Central retinal artery occlusion
What is Graves' disease?	The most common cause of hyperthyroidism. It is an autoimmune disease.
What is the treatment for Shigella?	Bactrim or fluoroquinolones and hydration
You hear a continuous machine-like murmur. What is the most likely diagnosis?	Patent ductus arteriosus (PDA)
At what age should a child begin to feed himself?	6 months
At what BMI should a patient be hospitalized for anorexia?	BMI of <17.5 or 20% below appropriate body weight

B

- A patient in the recovery room following foot surgery is complaining of severe photophobia. She feels as though there is something in her eye. What is the most likely diagnosis?

  Corneal abrasion (pt's scratch their eyes before they are completely awake from anesthesia)

- What organism is believed to be the main culprit in creating peptic ulcers?

  Helicobacter pylori

- What two lung cancers are typically found centrally on CXR?

  Small cell and squamous cell

- What is the best imaging to rule out testicular torsion?

  Doppler U/S for decreased blood flow to the testes

- Bloody stool with cysts and trophozoites should make you think of what diagnosis?

  Amebiasis

- How do you treat white oral plaques that can be scraped off?

  This is most likely candida. Topical nystatin or oral fluconazole 1 mg are first line choices.

- At approximately how many weeks pregnant is the uterus at the level of the symphysis pubis?

  12 weeks

- An abdominal exam with pain out of proportion to the exam should make you think of what diagnosis?

  Intestinal ischemia

- A 30 year old African American woman presents with dysphagia. You notice she also has thickened skin. A barium swallow demonstrates the absence of peristalsis. What is the most likely diagnosis?

  Scleroderma

- List three causes of decreased tactile fremitus.

  COPD, asthma, pleural effusion, pneumothorax

- How long must symptoms occur before diagnosing schizophrenia?

  At least six months

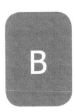

☐ Does total lung capacity go up or down in COPD?	*It goes up.*
☐ A positive Apley indicates what diagnosis?	*Meniscal tear*
☐ What is the first step in treating atopic dermatitis?	*Behavioral modifications - reduce bathing, only use soap on face and genitals, use natural breathable fabrics*
☐ Name one abortive drug for migraines.	*Triptans (sumatriptan, zolmitriptan), ergotamine*
☐ What is the most common microcytic anemia?	*Iron deficiency anemia*
☐ A biphasic P wave should make you think of what diagnosis?	*Left atrial enlargement*
☐ A cervical biopsy comes back as CIN1. What is the next step?	*Repeat pap smear in 6 months and repeat colposcopy in 12 months*
☐ A patient's mother has recommended that he see you. He lives on his own and is a computer programmer. He works from home. He has no friends and seldom leaves the house. She is concerned that he expresses no interest in meeting people and seems perfectly happy to be home alone all the time. What diagnosis should you be thinking of?	*Schizoid personality disorder*
☐ What is the medical term for tennis elbow?	*Lateral epicondylitis*
☐ What terms will likely be include in a description of a patient with a pheochromocytoma?	*Thin, diaphoretic, tachycardic, agitated*
☐ List three medication that may cause lupus.	*Procainamide, isoniazid and quinidine*
☐ A patient exhibits all of the characteristics of antisocial personality disorder, but he is only 14 years old. What diagnosis should you be thinking of?	*Conduct disorder*

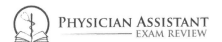

B

☐	What is the first line IV inotropic agent when dealing with cardiogenic shock?	*Dopamine*
☐	How long should pressure be applied to treat epistaxis?	*15 minutes*
☐	What is the gold standard for diagnosis and treatment of bile duct stones?	*ERCP*
☐	What is the most common cause of peptic ulcer disease?	*H. pylori*
☐	A child presents with painful ulcers in his mouth. On physical exam you find more of the same type of ulcers on his feet and hands. What virus is most likely causing these symptoms?	*Coxsackie virus*
☐	What medication is used to increase surfactant levels and help with lung maturity if you are worried about preterm labor?	*Betamethasone*
☐	List three medications which may be used for pharmacological stress test.	*Adenosine, dobutamine, dipyridamole and persantine*
☐	What is Trousseau's sign?	*Inflate BP cuff and hold for 3 minutes. Patient with low Ca will get carpel tunnel symptoms.*
☐	List the three cluster A personality disorders.	*"Mad" schizoid, schizotypal and paranoid*
☐	A palpable olive-shaped epigastric mass in a one month old should make you think of what diagnosis?	*Pyloric stenosis*
☐	What two leads do you use to determine the axis of the heart?	*Lead I and AVF*

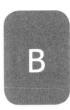

A study result comes back with intracellular neurofibrillary tangles and extracellular neuritic plaques. What diagnosis should you be thinking of?	Alzheimer's disease
What test do you do for Sjogren's syndrome?	Schirmer test
Will ACTH be elevated or decreased in Addison's disease?	Elevated if the problem is at the adrenal glands.
What are two medications used to induce labor?	Cervidil (Prostoglandin gel applied to the cervix) which encourages cervical ripening and oxytocin which encourages uterine contractions
Blue bloater refers to the characteristic physical exam findings of what disease?	Chronic bronchitis
Is an upper respiratory infection which includes hoarseness most likely bacterial or viral?	Viral
What is the time frame for the first symptoms of withdrawal from alcohol?	Tremor in 8-18 hrs
Tall peaked T waves should make you think of what diagnosis?	Hyperkalemia
A waxy stuck on appearance should make you think of what diagnosis?	Seborrheic keratosis
What is the initial treatment for a chemical burn to the eyes?	Irrigate, irrigate, irrigate
Are most pulmonary valve problems congenital or acquired?	95% are congenital
A patient is very concerned that she has breast cancer. In order to reassure her you perform a full workup which is negative. She is still unsatisfied and convinced that she has breast cancer. What diagnosis should you be thinking of?	Hypochondriasis

B

- Which anemia should you think of if you see the term Howell-Jolly bodies?

  Sickle cell due to the functional asplenia, but it may also show up in folic acid and B12 deficiency.

- What is the drug of choice to treat Lyme disease in kids or pregnant women?

  Amoxicillin

- What is the most common thyroid cancer?

  Papillary, makes up about 80% of thyroid cancers.

- List two medications you might use to treat an essential tremor.

  Beta blocker (propranolol), primidone

- What time frame are we talking about for chronic sinusitis?

  >3 months

- What is the most common cause of CHF?

  Coronary artery disease

- What will the bowel sounds be early on in a small bowel obstruction? What will they be later on?

  Early they are hyperactive. Late they are absent.

- Will a hemolytic anemia generally have an elevated or decreased retic count?

  Elevated

- What is the x-ray finding that supports diagnosis of a slipped capital femoral epiphysis?

  Ice cream falling of the cone

- What is the treatment for melanoma?

  Wide local excision

- How much fiber should you normally get in a day?

  About 30 grams

- A fundal exam shows a cherry-red spot. What is the most likely diagnosis?

  Central retinal artery occlusion

- Where are 90% of basal cell lesions found on the body?

  On the head and neck

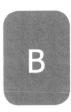

As part of the antepartum testing a baby has a positive stress test. What does that mean?	*They have had two heart rate accelerations in a 20 minute period of 15 beats above baseline for at least 15 seconds. This is a good thing.*
Define pellagra?	*Niacin (B3) deficiency*
List the 4 minor criteria for diagnosing endocarditis.	*Fever, embolic event (Janeway lesions or petechiae, splinter hemorrhages), immunological event (osler nodes, glomerulonephritis), 1 positive blood culture*
A 16 year old girl presents with an exudative sore throat and general malaise. On physical exam you observe some posterior chain lymphadenopathy and mild splenomegaly. What diagnosis should you be thinking of?	*Epstein–Barr virus*
What is the most common site of an ectopic pregnancy?	*Within a fallopian tube*
How do you treat achalasia?	*Loosen up the muscle - botox, dilation or surgery*
A CT scan of the head shows broad infiltration of orbital fat. What is the most likely diagnosis?	*Orbital cellulitis*
Zanamivir (Relenza) may be give to children above what age?	*7 years old*
List two macrolides.	*Erythromycin, azithromycin, clarithromycin*
What is the classic triad of pre-eclampsia?	*HTN, edema and proteinuria*
List the time of year when each of the following allergens is most prominent. Pollen, Grass, Ragweed and Mold.	*Pollen from trees and flowers = spring, grasses are the summer, mold and ragweed are fall*

B

☐	A wide pulse pressure with a blowing diastolic decrescendo murmur at the right 2nd intercostal space should make you think of what diagnosis?	*Aortic regurgitation*
☐	What class of antibiotics is sometimes prescribed specifically for its effects on increasing GI motility?	*Macrolides*
☐	What two labs do you want to monitor in a patient on an ACEI?	*Serum creatinine and serum potassium*
☐	At what age should a child be able to use a spoon and stack 3-4 blocks?	*18 months*
☐	A patient presents with acute swelling and pain in the cheek that increases at meals. What is the most likely diagnosis?	*Sialadenitis (salivary gland infection) - Staph aureus*
☐	What is the most common prophylactic antibiotic used preoperatively?	*Cefazolin = Ancef, Keflex = Cefalexin, The answer is Cefazolin (Ancef)*
☐	What is the most common organism causing pneumonia in COPD patients?	*Haemophilus influenzae*
☐	How do you treat amebiasis?	*Metronidazole (Flagyl)*
☐	What is another term for podagra?	*Gout*
☐	What is the most common cause of bronchiectasis?	*Cystic Fibrosis*
☐	According to the CDC, what is the range for a normal BMI?	*18.5-24.9*
☐	Colorectal cancer patients are almost all older than what age?	*90% of patients are older than 50.*
☐	What is the gold standard for diagnosing myocarditis?	*Myocardial biopsy*

B

List four complications of untreated strep throat.	*Scarlet fever, glomerulonephritis, rheumatic fever and local abscess*
Name three SSRI's.	*Fluoxetine, paroxetine, sertraline, citalopram, escitalopram, dapoxetine, zimelidine, mesembrine, seproxetine*
Duchenne's and Becker's muscular dystrophy have what genetic characteristic?	*X-linked recessive*
List the four cluster B personality disorders.	*"Bad" antisocial, borderline, histrionic and narcissistic*
If you come across a question where the patient has erythema nodosum and an enlarged parotid gland what diagnosis should you be thinking of?	*Sarcoidosis*
List 2 risk factors for ovarian cancer.	*BRCA1, family history, nulliparity, late menopause, Caucasian, Asian*
What happens to total lung capacity in sarcoidosis?	*It goes down.*
Where are Heberden's nodes found?	*Distal interphalangeal joint (DIP)*
What class of medications is the first line for lowering LDL?	*Statins*
Name two things that would constitute a positive stress test.	*A drop in blood pressure, a new arrhythmia, an increase in angina symptoms, ST depressions*
What is the average age of menopause?	*51*
What organism causes Lyme disease?	*Borrelia burgdorferi*
Give two contraindications for using an ACEI.	*Bilateral renal artery stenosis, history of angioedema, pregnancy*

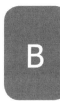

☐	Define the first stage of labor.	*Onset of contractions to full dilation of the cervix.*
☐	A sawtooth pattern on EKG should make you think of what diagnosis?	*Atrial flutter*
☐	A patient of Mediterranean descent is a clue for which type of anemia?	*Beta thalassemia*
☐	A patient having recently undergone cataract surgery presents complaining of vision loss in the operative eye. What diagnosis should you be thinking of?	*Retinal detachment*
☐	You suspect mitral regurgitation. What is the most accurate way to prove your diagnosis?	*Transesophageal echo*
☐	How do you administer the Rinne hearing test?	*Place the tuning fork on the mastoid and then move it next to the ear.*
☐	Ethambutol has what two major side effects?	*Optic neuritis, red green vision loss*
☐	What is the treatment for cholera?	*Fluids*
☐	Coal miners lung often shows nodular opacities in what lung fields?	*Upper lung fields*
☐	What is the first line antibiotic treatment for cystitis?	*Bactrim*
☐	What is the first line medical treatment for pericarditis?	*Aspirin and NSAIDS*
☐	Spaghetti and meatballs on KOH prep should make you think of what diagnosis?	*Tinea versicolor*
☐	Nummular eczema is most like what other dermatological disorder?	*Atopic dermatitis*

B

Is peptic ulcer disease more common in the duodenum or the stomach?	Duodenum
You suspect a pneumothorax. What instructions should go along with the order for a CXR?	It should be an end expiratory view in order to look for visceral pleural air.
A patient is very charming during his interview. You note during your interview that he has no concern for hurting or using other people. He seems to show no remorse for any of his actions. What diagnosis should you be thinking of?	Antisocial personality disorder
A patient presents with a round ulcer in her mouth that is yellow-grey and has a red halo. It is on the buccal mucosa and it is painful. What is the most likely diagnosis?	Aphthous ulcers
What are the most common colors lost in color blindness?	Red and green
A patient presents with erectile dysfunction and complains of some numbness in his feet. On second thought he has noticed significant polyuria and polydipsia. What diagnosis should you be thinking of?	Diabetic neuropathy
List the 5 insulins in order of peak efficacy?	Lispro 1-2 hrs, Regular 2-4 hrs, NPH 5-7 hrs, Lente 4-8 hrs, Ultralente 8-14 hrs.
A positive Hawkins test indicates what diagnosis?	Rotator cuff impingement
Which nerve root is responsible for the knee jerk reflex?	L3-L4
What are two common predisposing factors for esophageal varices?	Portal HTN and cirrhosis often caused by alcoholism.

B

☐	A patient presents with weakness that he has felt in his lower legs and now feels in his knees and hips bilaterally. He has decreased deep tendon reflexes. This has been getting progressively worse. What diagnosis should you be thinking of?	*Guillain-Barre*
☐	What are the two most common causes of epididymitis?	*Neisseria gonorrhea and chlamydia*
☐	Hampton's hump on CXR should make you think of what diagnosis?	*Pulmonary embolism*
☐	An African American female presents with malar rash and a positive double-stranded DNA antibody. What is the most likely diagnosis?	*Lupus*
☐	What is the most common knee injury?	*Medial meniscal tear*
☐	What is the term for difficulty swallowing?	*Dysphagia*
☐	List three side effects of digoxin.	*Nausea/vomiting, anorexia, confusion, arrhythmias (sinus brady, AV block), fatigue, vision disturbances etc.*
☐	Posturing should make you think of what diagnosis?	*Catatonic depression*
☐	Your attending asks you to come and see an excellent example of Hutchinson's sign. What diagnosis does the patient have?	*Herpes zoster ophthalmicus*
☐	What is the gold standard for diagnosing coronary artery disease?	*Cardiac catheterization*
☐	A 30 year old female presents with pustules on her face that spare the vermilion border. In her history she has been using topical steroids. What is the most likely diagnosis?	*Perioral dermatitis*

B

By what age should a child be able to hold up her head?	*3 months*
What is the term for being farsighted? What type of lens do you use to correct it?	*Hyperopia, convex*
Both testicles should be descended by what age?	*3 months*
What are two treatments you should consider for esophageal strictures?	*Dilation of the esophagus and long term PPIs*
Painless hematuria should make you think of what diagnosis?	*Bladder cancer*
What CXR finding might make you think of mesothelioma?	*Pleural thickening, remember 80% are found in the pleura lining*
Air fluid levels on abdominal x-ray should make you think of what diagnosis?	*Bowel obstruction*
You have a patient with diagnosis of a pheochromocytoma. While waiting for surgery, should you use an alpha blocker or a beta blocker?	*Alpha blocker. Never use a pure beta blocker.*
A patient being treated with penicillin for a syphilis infection develops fever, chills, muscle pain and headaches. Do you stop treatment?	*No this is Jarisch-Herxheimer reaction. The patient must be closely monitored, but it is a response to released endotoxin from the death of the spirochetes and not an allergic reaction.*
By what age should a child be able to walk?	*12 months*
When is watchful waiting with a diagnosis of acoustic neuroma an appropriate plan?	*This tumor is very slow growing. Watching a small tumor in an elderly patient is appropriate treatment.*
What is the treatment for Turner's syndrome?	*Cyclical estrogen and progesterone*

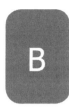

☐	What is the most common bladder cancer?	*Transitional cell cancer*
☐	A 4 year old boy presents between October and March with wheezing, coughing, a runny nose and increased respiratory rate. What is the most likely pathogen?	*Respiratory syncytial virus*
☐	What is the first line antibiotic for prostatitis?	*Bactrim 4-6 weeks*
☐	Does FEV1 go up or down with asthma?	*It goes down.*
☐	A patient exhibits splitting, seeing others as all good or all bad. What diagnosis should you be thinking of?	*Borderline personality disorder*
☐	A rope-like breast mass should make you think of what diagnosis?	*Fibrocystic breast mass*
☐	What is the most common primary intracranial neoplasm?	*Glioma*
☐	Name a common cause of a junctional rhythm.	*Digitoxin toxicity*
☐	A patient presents with unilateral hearing loss and a decrease in speech discrimination. She has also had difficulty with balance over the past week. What is the most likely diagnosis?	*Acoustic neuroma*
☐	You place a patient on rifampin. What side effect should you warn her about?	*Orange-red discoloration of body fluids*
☐	What specific breathing pattern is associated with diabetic ketoacidosis?	*Kussmaul respirations*
☐	What is the most common cause of sudden cardiac death?	*Ventricular fibrillation*
☐	When performing a decompression for a tension pneumothorax where do you put the needle?	*2nd intercostal space at the midclavicular line*

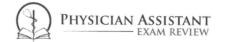

B

Is diphtheria a Gram-positive or negative organism?	Gram-positive
Patient presents with conjunctivitis, urethritis, arthritis and oral lesions. What is the most likely diagnosis? What other lab might you expect to be positive?	Reactive arthritis, HLA B-27
What is the name of the condition that involves fibrous scar tissue in the penis causing a curvature of the erect penis?	Peyronie's disease
What is the key indicator for the prognosis of melanoma?	Thickness of the lesion
What class of medications does pioglitazone (Actos) fall into?	Thiazolidinediones also known as glitazones
A patient's mother has recommended that he see you. He lives on his own and is a computer programmer. He works from home. He has no friends and seldom leaves the house. She is concerned that clearly he would like to meet people, but he is terrified of doing so. What diagnosis should you be thinking of?	Avoidant personality disorder
A lumbar puncture for a patient with bacterial meningitis will show elevated or decreased WBCs? Glucose? Protein?	Elevated WBCs, decreased glucose and elevated protein
A U wave on EKG should make you think of what diagnosis?	Hypokalemia
A patient presents with flaky skin in the nasolabial folds and on her scalp. What is the most likely diagnosis?	Seborrheic dermatitis
What is the most specific diagnostic test for peptic ulcer disease?	Endoscopy

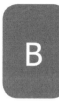

- Auer rods are most commonly associated with what disease? | Acute myeloid leukemia

- A positive McMurry indicates what diagnosis? | Meniscal tear

- What is the karyotype for a patient with Turner's syndrome? | (45, X) They are missing one sex chromosome.

- What is the most common location for a pancreatic tumor? | 75% occur in the head of the pancreas.

- What is the most specific imaging modality for diagnosing kidney stones? | CT

- A corkscrew appearance on barium study should make you think of what diagnosis? | Esophageal spasms

- What is the formula for calculating estimated date of confinement or due date? | First day of last menstrual period + 7 days - 3 months

- Name two tests you might use to rule out Cushing's syndrome. | 24 hour free cortisol urine test and dexamethasone suppression test

- If you have a patient with positive blood cultures for candida what is the first line drug? | Amphotericin B

- On physical exam, you notice ulnar deviations and swan neck deformities. What is the most likely diagnosis? | Rheumatoid arthritis

- A musical vibratory murmur best heard at the apex in a child should make you think of what diagnosis? | Still's murmur

- Pain with movement of the pinna or tragus should make you think of what diagnosis? | Otitis externa

- Small grouped vesicles on the vermillion border should make you think of what diagnosis? | Herpes

B

Define inevitable abortion.	*Vaginal bleeding, cervix is open, products of conception are still inside*
A patient presents with watery bilateral discharge from the eyes and nontender preauricular adenopathy. What is the most likely diagnosis? What is the most common pathogen?	*Viral conjunctivitis, adenovirus*
A barrel chest should make you think of what diagnosis?	*Emphysema*
What does Kiesselbach's plexus refer to?	*A group of vein's in the anterior nose which bleed a lot.*
A woman presents to the ER concerned she is in preterm labor. What treatment should you begin before even getting any imaging or lab results?	*Give IV fluids (most often the patient is suffereing from dehydration)*
A college student presents with a little purulent drainage from one eye and nontender preauricular lymphadenopathy. What diagnosis and pathogen should you be thinking of?	*Chlamydia conjunctivitis*
What is the treatment for seborrheic keratosis?	*It is bengin so there is no need to treat it. Lesions may be removed if unsightly.*
Are ulcers from venous insufficiency painful or painless?	*Painless*
A 95 year old female presents to ER after a fall in her home. Her left leg is shortened and externally rotated. What is the most likely diagnosis?	*Hip fracture*
Giant cell arteritis is associated with what other disease?	*Polymyalgia rheumatica*
Elevated circulating acetylcholine receptor antibodies should make you think of what diagnosis?	*Myasthenia gravis*

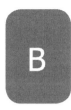

☐ What is the suffix associated with sulfonylureas?	*ide is the suffix. Examples are glipizide, tolbutamide, tolazamide.*
☐ A patient presents complaining of a metallic taste in her mouth and dark brown urine. What antibiotic might she be on?	*Metronidazole (Flagyl)*
☐ What will an x-ray show in acute osteomyelitis?	*Nothing - it will show bone destruction in chronic osteomyelitis.*
☐ What two psychiatric issues are more common in males than females?	*Autism and ADD, the rest are all either equal or more common in females.*
☐ What does ERCP stand for?	*Endoscopic retrograde cholangiopancreatography*
☐ Define abortion.	*Delivery of uterine contents before 20 weeks.*
☐ A COPD patient has apical cavities and calcified nodes on his CXR. You also discover he has a pet bat and a few birds. What diagnosis should you be thinking of?	*Histoplasmosis*
☐ Does an increase in reticulocytes indicate a decrease or an increase in RBC production?	*An increase, reticulocytes are newly released "baby" RBC's*
☐ A young boy comes into your office. He has elevated blood pressure when taken in his arm, but no femoral pulses can be palpated. What is the most likely diagnosis?	*Coarctation of the aorta*
☐ A patient presents with mucopurulent discharge and cervical motion tenderness. What is the most likely diagnosis?	*Chlamydia - cervicitis*
☐ A patient presents with acute onset of continuous severe vertigo for the past five days. He does have a history of URI 2 weeks ago. What is the most likely diagnosis?	*Labrynthitis*

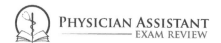

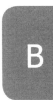

☐	What is the best test to check for H. pylori?	*Urea breath test*
☐	What is the most common cause of an upper respiratory tract infection?	*Rhinovirus*
☐	A patient presents with inability to speak and right sided weakness. He seems to understand speech and follows commands well. What type of aphasia should you be thinking of?	*Broca's aphasia*
☐	What is the best lab test for scabies?	*Microscopic examination under oil immersion*
☐	A stuck on grey membrane in the pharynx should make you think of what diagnosis?	*Diphtheria*
☐	A patient recently started taking Lipitor. He is now complaining of aches and pains. What test should you order?	*Serum creatinine kinase, you're looking for rhabdomyolysis*
☐	Which cardiac medication has gynecomastia in its side effect profile?	*Spironolactone*
☐	What will the likely findings be on a CXR of a patient with asbestosis?	*Linear opacities at the bases with pleural plaques*
☐	What is the medication of choice for a patient with Tourette's syndrome?	*Haloperidol*
☐	A positive Phalen and Tinel's sign indicates what diagnosis?	*Carpal tunnel*
☐	Lead pipe or cogwheel rigidity should make you think of what diagnosis?	*Parkinson's disease*
☐	A 5 year old presents in early January with a red itchy rash behind his knees. You notice it on the flexor surfaces of his elbows as well. What is the most likely diagnosis?	*Atopic dermatitis*

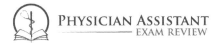

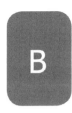

☐ At what age should you begin ordering dexa scans for male patients? What about female patients?	70 for males, 65 for females
☐ What is the condition where the urethral meatus is not at the tip of the penis?	Hypospadias and in far fewer cases epispadias.
☐ A Gram-positive organism in chains should make you think of what diagnosis?	Strep
☐ Which reproductive cancer carries the highest rates of death in women?	Ovarian cancer
☐ A slowly growing nodule with a central depression and a pearly border should make you think of what diagnosis?	Basal cell carcinoma
☐ What is the imaging modality of choice for pancreatitis?	CT
☐ During pregnancy which is the prefered treatment of hyperthyroidism PTU or methimazole?	PTU
☐ What is the hallmark physical exam finding for placenta previa?	Trick question - NEVER do a physical exam on someone with presumed placenta previa.
☐ What is the first line medication for a patient with symptomatic bradycardia?	Atropine
☐ Is a nulliparous or mulitparous woman more likely to get preeclampsia?	Nulliparity is a risk factor for preeclampsia.
☐ What medication is a good place to start treating bipolar 1 or 2?	Lithium
☐ Any question about rabbits and pneumonia should make you think of what diagnosis?	Tularemia

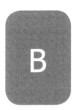

On EKG there is an early but otherwise normal PQRS complex. After that beat there is a slight pause and then a normal rhythm continues. What is the term for this one beat?	*Premature atrial contraction*
A patient presents to the ER in acute CHF. What drug class will likely be the first choice?	*Loop diuretics*
A college student presents with copious purulent drainage from one eye. What diagnosis and pathogen should you be thinking of?	*Neisseria conjunctivitis*
What are the ABC's of melanoma?	*Asymmetry, border, color, diameter, elevation/irregularity, evolving*
Honey and babies should make you think of what diagnosis?	*Botulism*
How long must symptoms last before diagnosing ADD?	*6 months*
Should diverticulitis always be admitted?	*No, mild cases can be treated as outpatients with rest and clear fluids.*
You hear a loud, harsh pulmonary murmur along the left sternal border. What is the most likely diagnosis?	*Ventricular septal defect*
What is Charcot's triad?	*RUQ pain, fever, jaundice*
What percentage of diabetes in the US is type 2?	*80-90%*
Paroxysmal nocturnal dyspnea should make you think of what diagnosis?	*CHF*
Describe Brudzinski's sign.	*When you lift the patient's head the patient bends his hips.*

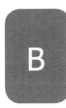

☐	What is the most common place for an aortic aneurysm?	*In the abdomen and below the renal arteries*
☐	Why aren't fluoroquinolones used more frequently?	*They have lots of side effects.*
☐	What is the first step in treating GERD?	*Lifestyle modification*
☐	A shuffling gait should make you think of what diagnosis?	*Parkinson's disease*
☐	Is FSH high or low in Turner's syndrome?	*High, there are no ovaries to respond to FSH and so there is no negative feedback*
☐	What location within the pelvis is endometriosis most commonly found?	*On an ovary.*
☐	How is the first day of the menstrual cycle defined?	*The first day of menstrual bleeding is the first day of the cycle.*
☐	A patient presents complaining of right upper quadrant pain 20 minutes after meals. What is the most likely diagnosis?	*Cholecystitis*
☐	There is an MRI result of multiple foci of demyelination in the white matter. What diagnosis should you be thinking of?	*Multiple sclerosis*
☐	What is Sheehan's syndrome?	*Ischemia of the pituitary due to volume depletion during or after childbirth.*
☐	What is the gold standard for diagnosis of giant cell arteritis?	*Biopsy of the temporal artery*
☐	What medication is used as prophylaxis for meningococcal meningits?	*Rifampin*
☐	What is the medical term for hunchback?	*Kyphosis*

B

How do you test for color blindness?	*Ishihara plates*
How often should a diabetic's HgbA1c be checked and what should it be?	*Every three months (remember the life of an RBC is 90-120 days) and it should be below 6.5%.*
A pathology report comes back showing negatively birefringent crystals. What is the most likely diagnosis?	*Gout*
What is the normal pH of the blood?	*7.35-7.45*
An RSR prime in leads V1 or V2 should make you think of what diagnosis?	*Right bundle branch block*
What is the appropriate treatment for a patent ductus arteriosus.	*Indomethacin*
What is the major concern with using lithium?	*It has a very narrow therapeutic window. Blood tests are needed every four weeks.*
List three risk factors for placental abruption.	*HTN, smoking, AMA, cocaine use, PROM*
Would a B12 deficiency anemia most likely be microcytic, normocytic or macrocytic?	*Macrocytic*
What is the term for eyelids that turn out?	*Ectropion*
Are one half of all adult hernias direct or indirect inguinal hernias?	*Indirect inguinal hernias makeup 50% of all adult hernias.*
Will the serum ferritin be high or low in a patient with iron deficient anemia?	*It will almost always be low.*
A patient has a silver-fork deformity on x-ray. What is the most likely diagnosis?	*Colles fracture*

B

☐ What is the first line treatment for carpal tunnel?	*Night splint*
☐ Define procidentia.	*Uterine prolapse beyond the introitus.*
☐ What is the most important complication of giant cell arteritis?	*Blindness*
☐ List 4 medications which may cause asthma.	*Beta blockers, NSAIDS, ACEI, ASA*
☐ A fat pad sign on a lateral x-ray of the elbow has what significance?	*It is blood in the joint indicating a fracture even if the fracture line cannot be seen.*
☐ A PSA above what level should start to make you concerned?	*>4.0*
☐ At what age do symptoms of Huntington's disease appear?	*Around 30 years old*
☐ Bird-beak esophagus on barium swallow should make you think of what diagnosis?	*Achalasia*
☐ What is the suffix for used for most fluoroquinolones?	*Oxacin*
☐ List six extrapulmonary complications of lung cancer.	*SPHERE - SVC syndrome, Pancoast tumor, Horner's syndrome, Endocrine problems, Recurrent laryngeal symptoms, Effusions (exudative)*
☐ During an interview a patient states "I have been anxious for as long as I can remember." This statement should make you think of what diagnosis?	*Generalized anxiety disorder*
☐ A patient presents to the ER with chest pain. An EKG shows diffuse ST elevations in almost all of the leads. What is the most likely diagnosis?	*Pericarditis*

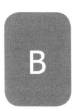

During a physical exam of a child, you feel a tubular or sausage-shaped mass. What diagnosis should you be thinking of?	*Intussusception*
A Salter-Harris type III fracture affects what area of the bone?	*The physis (growth plate) as well as the epiphysis.*
An ovarian cyst that contains hair and teeth should make you think of what diagnosis?	*Teratoma*
A 34 year old presents with symptoms which are relapsing and remitting over the past few weeks. These include visual problems and weakness in her right arm. What is the most likely diagnosis?	*Multiple sclerosis*
List two risk factors for cervical cancer.	*Multiple sexual partners, smoking*
What is the most common type of kidney stone?	*Calcium makes up 85% of kidney stones.*
You recommend bisphosphonates for a patient with osteoporosis. What instruction do you give her for immediately after taking the medication?	*Remain upright for 30 minutes*
Give two major risk factors for erectile dysfunction.	*Diabetes, hypertension, depression, coronary artery disease*
You believe a patient has had a stroke. He presents with aphasia, loss of hearing in one ear and loss of vision in his left eye. Is the blockage likely in the anterior or posterior circulation?	*Anterior*
What hereditary pattern does polycystic kidney disease follow?	*Autosomal dominant*
What is the treatment for giant cell arteritis?	*High dose prednisone*

B

Wilson's disease is associated with a build up of what mineral?	*There is a deficiency of the copper binding protein and therefore a buildup of copper.*
What is the treatment for epididymitis?	*Ceftriaxone and doxycycline*
A child with bulky greasy stool should make you think of what diagnosis?	*Cystic fibrosis*
A christmas tree pattern should make you think of what diagnosis?	*Pityriasis rosea*
How do you treat urethritis?	*Ceftriaxone and doxycycline*
What organism is the most common cause of pneumonia in a patient with cystic fibrosis?	*Pseudomonas*
Where is disease of the tricuspid valve best heard?	*Along the left lower sternal border.*
A positive Finkelstein's test indicates what diagnosis?	*de Quervain's tenosynovitis*
How do you treat dyshidrosis?	*Topical steroids*
What are the genetic characteristics of Wilson's disease?	*Autosomal recessive, chromosome 13*
A question stem includes an IV drug user with a new heart murmur and fever. What is the most likely diagnosis?	*Endocarditis*
What will a CXR show for a patient with an aortic dissection?	*Widened mediastinum*
Are patients with specific phobias aware they are strange?	*Yes*

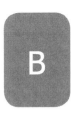

What antibiotic is the first line treatment for mycoplasma pneumonia?	A macrolide, erythromycin or azithromycin
What is the first step of treatment for endometrial cancer?	Total hysterectomy and bilateral salpingo-oophorectomy
Name three medication "classes" which are used to reduce LDL?	Statins, ezetimibe, niacin and nicotinic acid
What is the prophylactic antibiotic most commonly given before a dental procedure if one is necessary?	Amoxicillin 2 grams po 1 hour before procedure
A patient was in the woods yesterday and today presents with erythema migrans. What diagnosis should you be thinking of?	Lyme disease
Iron deficiency anemia will have a serum iron lower than what value?	30
Which way does a Colles fracture angulate: dorsal or volar? What about a Smith fracture?	Colles = Dorsal, Smith = Volar
What is the term for being nearsighted? What type of lens do you use to correct it?	Myopia, concave lenses
A urine protein of >3.5 grams/day should make you think of what diagnosis?	Nephrotic syndrome
What is the most common cause of subarachnoid hemorrhage aside from trauma?	Ruptured cerebral aneurysm
What type of incontinence is often associated with BPH?	Overflow incontinence, the bladder cannot empty sufficiently
If you believe there may be a foreign body obstructing a child's breathing what type of CXR should you order?	Expiratory view looking for hyperinflation due to air trapping.

B

A 66 year old female patient presents with bouts of nausea, weight loss and vague abdominal pain. What is the most likely diagnosis?	Ovarian cancer
Currant jelly stool should make you think of what diagnosis?	Intussusception
What is the best imaging to diagnose osteomyelitis?	Bone scan or MRI
Why is folic acid given as a prenatal vitamin?	Low folic acid can lead to neural tube defects.
Imaging is negative for blood, but you strongly believe that there is a subarachnoid hemorrhage. What test can you order that will be definitive?	Lumbar puncture
What is the treatment for pneumocystis jiroveci pneumonia?	Bactrim
Describe Barlow's test.	Adduct and internal rotation of the hips
A 19 year old male took an elbow to the face while playing basketball this morning. The whole left side of his face is swollen and he can't look up. What is the most likely diagnosis?	Orbital fracture
Following a myocardial infarction, what medication should you be using to treat hypertension?	Beta blocker
Borderline personality disorder is on the border of what two psychological disorders?	Neurosis and psychosis
Give the dexa score for osteopenia and osteoporosis.	Osteopenia = 1 to 2.4 standard deviations, osteoporosis = 2.5 standard deviations or greater

B

A patient complains of pain in his legs when he walks. It goes away after sitting. What term comes to mind for this symptom? What diagnosis is it associated with?	Intermittent claudication caused by peripheral arterial disease.
What is the most common infection following a C-section?	Metritis
Which medication is worse to give to a pediatric patient, tetracycline or an aminoglycoside?	Tetracycline
What is the term for when the placenta has implanted directly over the cervical os?	Placenta previa
A patient is arrogant with an inflated self image. He feels he is special and should be treated that way. What diagnosis should you be thinking of?	Narcissistic personality disorder
Often caused by chlamydia what is the syndrome characterized by urethritis (or cervicitis), arthritis and conjuctivitis?	Reiter's syndrome
What is the drug of choice for treating Rocky Mountain spotted fever?	Doxycycline
What tumor marker can be used to follow pancreatic cancer?	CA-19-9
What is the most common cause of hyperparathyroidism?	Single parathyroid adenoma in 80% of cases.
A patient has very strange magical thinking. What diagnosis should you be thinking of?	Schizotypal personality disorder
Will the retic count be elevated, decreased or normal in a B12 deficient anemia?	Retic count will be low. Low building blocks means low production.

B

A patient presents with a painful ipsilateral third nerve palsy. What diagnosis should you be thinking of?	Posterior communicating artery aneurysm (PComA)
Does mastitis tend to be unilateral or bilateral?	Unilateral and only one quadrant
What is the name for the triangular or wedge shaped growth on the conjunctiva that may interfere with vision?	Pterygium
A college student presents with pneumonia. What two organisms should you be thinking of?	Chlamydia and mycoplasma
What is the most common cause of acute bacterial cholangitis?	Choledocholithiasis
A patient complains of severe crushing chest pain. EKG shows ST segment elevations. All labs including troponins and CK-MB are negative. What is the most likely diagnosis?	Prinzmetal's angina
Vision loss described as a curtain coming down should make you think of what diagnosis?	Retinal detachment
What is the initial treatment for active TB?	INH+RIF+PZA+EMB x several months typically followed by INH+RIF once sensativities come back.
What ethnic background is at an increased risk of fibroids?	African Americans are 5x more likely to have fibroids compared to Caucasian women.
Name the condition in which the head of the penis curves downward or upward, at the junction of the head and shaft of the penis. (Hint: It is often associated with hypospadias.)	Chordee
Will a spermatocele transillumnate?	Yes

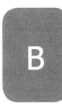

A psychiatric patient presents with confusion, fever and lead pipe rigidity. What diagnosis should you be thinking of?	Neuroleptic malignant syndrome, this can occur with high dose antipsychotics.
A patient expresses concern that he can't trust anyone. That everyone is out to get him, and his problems are all the faults of others. He has held very long grudges due to perceived past wrongs. What diagnosis should you be thinking of?	Paranoid personality disorder
What is the treatment of choice for strep throat?	Penicllin, amoxicillin, erythromycin
On EKG, there is an early wide QRS complex with no associated P wave. After that beat, there is a slight pause, and then a normal rhythm continues. What is the term for this one beat?	Premature ventricular contraction
A feathery border in an eye exam should make you think of what diagnosis?	Fungal infection
On palpation, what size is normal for the aorta?	Less than 3 cm
What occupations are associated with berylliosis?	Aerospace and nuclear plant workers
During what portion of the menstrual cycle does PMS occur?	By definition it is in the second half and menstruation should relieve the symptoms.
What is the test to begin with if you suspect a pheochromocytoma?	24 hour urine for catecholamines
A beta natriuretic peptide below what level rules out CHF?	<100
What it is the recommended treatment for hepatitis C infection?	Pegylated interferon alpha-2
An Osborn or J wave on EKG should make you think of what diagnosis?	Hypothermia

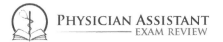

B

What is the first symptom of a rabies infection?	Pain and anesthesia at the site of the bite
Tea-colored urine with red cell casts should make you think of what diagnosis?	Glomerulonephritis
A doughnut shaped burn should make you think of what issue?	Abuse, either child or elder
A gastrinoma is also known as what syndrome?	Zollinger-Ellison syndrome
You have a patient with major depressive disorder. Once his symptoms have completely resolved how long should you continue with treatment?	A six month minimum is recomended due to very high relapse rates.
A child presents with paroxysmal abdominal pain, nausea, vomiting and diarrhea. What diagnosis should you be thinking of?	Intussusception
About how much weight should a woman gain during pregnancy?	20-35 lbs
Is metformin indicated or contraindicated in renal failure?	Contraindicated
The secretory phase of the mestraul cycle (day 14-28) is dominated by what hormone?	Progesterone
Name one oral medication that can be used for MRSA.	Linezolid (Zyvox) and Bactrim
What causes anorexic patients to have osteopenia?	A decrease in estrogen
The follicular phase of menstruation is dominated by what hormone?	Estrogen
What causes Mallory-Weiss tears?	Forced vomiting or retching (often involving alcohol)

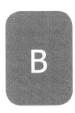

List the two cluster C personality disorders.	"Sad" avoidant and obsessive compulsive
An RSR prime in leads V5 or V6 should make you think of what diagnosis?	Left bundle branch block
White blood cell casts should make you think of what diagnosis?	Pyelonephritis
Does a patient with mitral valve prolapse require prophylactic antibiotics for dental work?	No, a recent change moves mitral valve prolapse from high risk to moderate risk.
What will the heart rate be if the AV node is pacing the heart?	40-60 beats per minute
Under routine circumstances when should patients begin getting screening colonoscopies?	Age 50
A Blalock procedure is used to correct what congenital heart condition?	Tetralogy of Fallot
Under what conditions would aspirin or clopidogrel be used following a TIA as prophylaxis?	These are antiplatelet medications. They would be used unless there is a known cardiac etiology for the embolism. Patients with a cardiac cause should use heparin or Coumadin.
What is the best test for diagnosing CHF?	Echo
A positive crossover test indicates what diagnosis?	Acromioclavicular joint injury (AC joint)
What tests are done to screen for HIV?	ELISA, then if positive the diagnosis is confirmed with a Western blot test.
Is Klebsiella gram (+) or gram (-)?	Gram (-)

B

What organism causes us to warn pregnant patients to stay away from deli meats and soft cheeses?	Listeria
What is the first line treatment for mastitis?	Dicloxacillin is first line. Cephalexin or erythromycin are second line.
What is the #1 cause of septic arthritis in sexually active young adults?	Neisseria gonorrhoeae
What is the normal level of serum bicarbonate (HCO3)?	24 mEq/Liter
Feeling a bag of worms in the scrotum should make you think of what diagnosis?	Varicocele
Epigastric abdominal pain which radiates to the back should make you think of what diagnosis?	Pancreatitis
A patient who has normal bladder function, but can not get to the bathroom has what type of incontinence?	Functional incontinence
A patient presents with unilateral blurriness developing over a few days. Fundal exam shows a "blood and thunder" pattern. What diagnosis should you be thinking of?	Central vein occlusion
What is the best test to diagnose an aortic dissection?	CT
A Gram-negative coccobaccili found in the sputum of patient with pneumonia should make you think of what diagonsis?	H. flu
A question about Prinzmetal's angina will often contain what key thing in the patient's history?	Cocaine use

B

What antibiotic class is the class of choice for chlamydia?	Macrolides
A patient with rheumatoid arthritis is heading to the OR for open reduction and internal fixation of the ankle. In addition to ankle films, what other x-rays should you get?	C-spine, anesthesia will want them due to concerns about instability of C1 & C2.
A lacey pink rash on the face of a child should make you think of what diagnosis?	Erythema infectiosum aka fifth disease aka slapped cheek
A patient presents to the ER with saddle anesthesia and loss of bowel and bladder function. What is the most likely diagnosis?	Cauda equina
What are the three most common cancers to metastasize to the lungs?	Breast, liver and colon
What is a cystocele?	A herniation of the bladder into the vagina.
Will evidence of TB be seen more frequently in the upper or lower lung lobes on CXR?	Upper
An older patient presents with pneumonia and diarrhea. What diagnosis should you be thinking of?	Legionella pneumonia
What is considered a normal PCO2?	40mmHG
How do you treat a Trichomonas infection?	Metronidazole
What is the most common organism responsible for prostatitis?	E. coli
List two risk factors for an aortic dissection?	Hypertension, Marfan's syndrome, bicuspid aortic valve, pregnancy

B

A fixed or consistent split S2 should make you think of what diagnosis?	Atrial septal defect
Describe Courvoisier's sign.	Nontender, palpable gallbladder which may indicate pancreatic neoplasm.
A patient presents saying that he doesn't seem to need his glasses anymore after 30 yrs. What is the most likely diagnosis?	Cataract
What life threatening side effect do statins have?	Rhabdomyolysis
What medication is most commonly used for long term treatment of GERD?	Proton pump inhibitors - omeprazole, lansoprazole, pantoprazole
A boot-shaped heart on CXR should make you think of what congenital heart condition?	Tetralogy of Fallot
By what age should a child be able to sit up?	6 months
Stocking glove anesthesia should make you think of what diagnosis?	Diabetic neuropathy and B12 deficiency neuropathy
What is the treatment goal for a diabetic with hypertension?	130/80
If you see a question with an alcoholic who has been diagnosed with pneumonia what is the most likely organism?	Klebsiella pneumoniae
You see regular P waves and regular QRS complexes, but they do not seem to have any correlation to each other. What is the diagnosis?	Third degree AV block
A 6 year old boy seems to have all of the symptoms of ADD while at school, but at home he has no problems. Does he have ADD?	No, symptoms must occur in both settings for diagnosis.

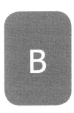

Name the sign which is defined as decreased pain with scrotal elevation?	Prehn's sign
A patient complains of an aching headache which feels like a band around his head. What diagnosis should you be thinking of?	Tension headache
Waxy flexibility should make you think of what diagnosis?	Catatonic schizophrenia
A thumbprint sign on x-ray should make you think of what two diagnoses?	Lateral C-spine = epiglottitis, abdominal = intestinal ischemia
A noncaseating granuloma should make you think of what diagnosis?	Sarcoidosis
List the six P's of an ischemic limb.	Pain, paresthesias, pallor, pulselessness, poikilothermia, paralysis
A pathology report comes back with positive birefringent crystals. What is the most likely diagnosis?	Pseudogout
What medication is often used to treat postpartum depression in a woman who is breast feeding?	Sertraline (Zoloft)
A thin looking heart and flattened diaphragm on CXR should make you think of what diagnosis?	Emphysema
A diaper rash with satellite lesions should make you think of what diagnosis?	Candida
Name the four thyroid cancers.	Papillary, Follicular, Medullary, Anaplastic
There are vaccines for which two versions of hepatitis?	Hepatitis A and hepatitis B

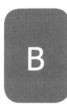

☐ Describe Kernig's sign.	*The patient lies supine, flex hip while keeping knee straight. Back pain is positive.*
☐ Which nerve is involved in herpes zoster ophthalmicus?	*Trigeminal nerve, CN 5*
☐ Hyperpigmented velvety plaques should make you think of what diagnosis?	*Acanthosis nigricans*
☐ Oseltamivir (Tamiflu) may be given to children above what age?	*1 year old*
☐ What is the gold standard for diagnosis of a pleural effusion?	*Thoracocentesis*
☐ What is the most common organism that causes a bladder infection?	*E. coli*
☐ Interference with work or school is part of which diagnosis, premenstrual syndrome or premenstrual dysphoric disorder?	*Premenstrual dysphoric disorder*
☐ Giant cells on a Tzanck smear should make you think of what diagnosis?	*Herpes simplex virus*
☐ A patient ate out last night and today has cramping and bloody diarrhea. What is the most likely organism?	*Salmonella*
☐ What symptom is associated with a classic migraine?	*Having an aura*
☐ What are the 5 criteria for metabolic syndrome?	*HDL <40 men <50 females, BP >135/85, Triglycerides >150, Fasting glucose >100, Waist >40 inches in men >35 inches in women*

B

What is the drug of choice for the treatment of syphilis?	Pencillin
The baby was delivered several minutes ago. Suddenly there is a increase in blood flow from the vagina and the cord noticeably lengthens. What is the most likely cause of these signs?	Placental separation
What is Russell's sign?	Abraded knuckles from forcing oneself to vomit.
What is the best test to diagnose bronchiectasis?	CT
A surge in what hormone leads to ovulation?	Luteinizing hormone (LH)
What are two important things you need to tell you patients before putting them on metronidazole?	Stay out of the sun and avoid alcohol.
An EEG showing interictal spikes should make you think of what diagnosis?	Complex partial seizure
Which EKG leads are used to diagnose an anterior wall MI?	V1, V2 and V3
A new mother presents with pain over the radial wrist. She has a positive Finkelstein's test. What is the most likely diagnosis?	de Quervain's tenosynovitis
What would you expect the WBC count to be in the joint fluid of an infected knee?	>50,000 at a minimum and probably much higher.
A blockage of which artery causes a lateral wall MI?	Left circumflex artery
Posttussive rales should make you think of what diagnosis?	TB
Statins are the drug of choice to treat what type of dyslipidemia?	Elevated LDL

B

☐ Where is a Pancoast tumor found on CXR?	At the apex of either the right or left lung
☐ An epigastric olive-shaped mass should make you think of what diagnosis?	Pyloric stenosis
☐ Pertussis is most commonly treated with what antibiotic?	Erythromycin
☐ Forchheimer spots are associated with what disease?	Rubella
☐ Define complete abortion.	Vaginal bleeding, cervix open, products of conception have passed
☐ How do fibrates work to affect the lipid profile?	They inhibit synthesis of VLDL and elevate lipoprotein lipase.
☐ What is the most common way of testing for metamorphopsia?	Amsler grid
☐ A contralateral mediastinal shift should make you think of what diagnosis?	Tension pneumothorax
☐ What drug is used for the treatment or prophylaxis of malaria?	Chloroquine
☐ A white oral lesion which cannot be scraped off should make you think of what diagnosis?	Oral leukoplakia
☐ What are the three inferior leads?	II, III and aVF
☐ Which cardiac medication is used to help with cardiac contractility after you have optimized most of the other cardiac medications?	Digoxin
☐ Describe Cullen's sign.	Umbilical ecchymosis often related to pancreatitis.

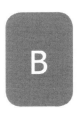

☐	What is the therapeutic range for INR following a mechanical valve replacement?	2.5-3.5
☐	A patient has an intracranial neoplasm causing auditory illusions, olfactory hallucinations and emotional changes. What lobe is the lesion likely in?	Temporal
☐	Give two risk factors for glaucoma.	African American decent and diabetes
☐	The EKG shows irregularly irregular narrow QRS waves. What is the most likely diagnosis?	Atrial fibrillation
☐	A patient presents with a ruptured Achilles tendon. He states he that he was recently in the hospital for a "blood infection and on a ton of antibiotics." What antibiotic class may he have been on?	Fluoroquinolones
☐	A patient with a history of hepatitis B presents complaning of bilateral knee pain, fever and weight loss. What is the most likely diagnosis?	Polyarteritis nodosa
☐	A physical exam finding of egophony should make you think of what diagonsis?	Lobar pneumonia
☐	Prolonged expiration (low FFV1) should make you think of what diagnosis?	Asthma or COPD
☐	Anatomically where are 80% of clavicle fractures located?	Middle third
☐	What is the first line of treatment for an anal fissure?	Fluid and fiber
☐	No matter what medications you use you are having trouble keeping a patient's blood pressure under control. You also notice hyperpigmented skin and truncal obesity. What is the most likely diagnosis?	Cushing's disease
☐	What is the best location to hear problems with the aortic valve?	2nd right intercostal space

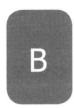

☐ What medication(s) are used to treat a postpartum metritis?	*Clindamycin and gentamicin together*
☐ If a question presents a pregnant woman with anemia what is the most likely diagnosis?	*Iron deficiency*
☐ Define premature birth.	*Delivery before 37 weeks.*
☐ Why is ovarian cancer so hard to diagnosis?	*There are no good markers and the symptoms are very vague.*
☐ You feel a pulse that seems to be vibrating. What term do you use to describe it?	*Thrill*
☐ List six medications that can be used for migraine prophylaxis?	*Beta blockers, tricyclics, calcium channel blockers, NSAIDs and valproic acid*
☐ At what age is primary amenorrhea diagnosed?	*Age 14 if no secondary sex characteristics. Age 16 if some secondary development.*
☐ Describe the pattern of weight gain in an infant over the following time periods: week one, 6 months, 12 months, 3 years old and 4 years old.	*Newborns lose 10% of their birth weight initially but are back to birth weight at 10 days, 6m = 2x birth weight, 12m = 3x birthweight, 3 y/o= 30 lbs & 30 inches, 4 y/o = 40 lbs & 40 inches*
☐ What is the most likely quadrant for a retinal detachment?	*Superior temporal*
☐ At what percentage of blockage is an endarterectomy indicated?	*Asymptomatic >70%, symptomatic >60%*
☐ What ligament is most commonly injured in an ankle sprain?	*Anterior talofibular ligament (ATFL)*

B

What is the medical term for feeling like there is a lump in your throat?	Globus
A strawberry cervix with copious yellow/green discharge should make you think of what diagnosis?	Trichomonas vaginitis
What two blood test can be used to diagnose celiac?	IgA endomysial antibody and IgA tTG antibody
What type of mosquitoes carry malaria?	Anopheles
A CXR shows vascular redistribution and blurred vascular outlines. What is the most likely diagnosis?	CHF
An EKG shows a regular heart rate of 200 bpms. QRS is narrow. What is the most likely diagnosis?	Supraventricular tachycardia
Where is disease of the mitral valve best heard?	At the apex
Transudative pleural effusions should make you think of what diagnosis?	Congestive heart failure
A slit lamp shows Kayser-Fleischer rings. What diagnosis should you be thinking of?	Wilson's disease
Where are Bouchard's nodes found?	Proximal interphalangeal joint (PIP)
At approximately how many weeks pregnant is the uterus at the level of the umbilicus?	20 weeks
What is the medical term for golfer's elbow?	Medial epicondylitis
What organism is the most common cause of an uncomplicated urinary tract infection?	E. Coli

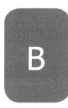

☐ A 15 year old overweight boy presents to your office limping with knee pain. What is the most likely diagnosis?	*Slipped capital femoral epiphysis*
☐ What Rh combination for mom and dad might cause the mother to create antiboides against the baby's red blood cells?	*Mom Rh-negative and dad Rh-positive*
☐ What are the two important peices of patient education for anyone diagnosed with mononucleosis?	*No contact sports (splenic rupture) and no kissing (highly contagious)*
☐ What is the leading cause of iron deficiency anemia?	*Chronic GI bleed*
☐ How do hookworm larvae enter the body?	*They penetrate the skin usually through the soles of the feet.*
☐ What four chromosomes have been linked to dementia?	*1,14,19,21*
☐ Clot busting drugs should be used within 3 hours of which two cardiac events?	*STEMI and new left bundle branch block*
☐ What is the medical treatment for gout?	*Allopurinol, colchicine*
☐ How do sulfonylureas work?	*They stimulate the production of insulin.*
☐ At what age do you begin screening patients for prostate cancer? What two tests are used?	*At age 50 an annual digital rectal exam and a PSA are recommended.*
☐ Define pulsus alternans.	*EKG waveform changes from beat to beat.*
☐ Melasma is most often found in what patient population?	*Women of childbearing age*
☐ What is the first line treatment for tinea corporis?	*Topical azoles*

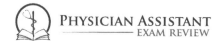

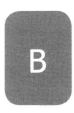

What organism is the most common cause of otitis media?	Strep pneumonia
Salivary amylase breaks down what macronutrient?	Carbohydrates
What dermatologic finding is associated with asthma?	Atopic dermatitis
How long after administering a PPD should it be read?	48-72 hours
What is the treatment for ovarian cancer?	Total hysterectomy and bilateral salpingo-oophorectomy. Then chemo and radiation.
How do glitazones work?	They improve insulin sensitivity
What is the best test to diagnose malaria?	Peripheral blood smear
A premature infant with hyaline membrane disease will have what appearance on CXR?	Bilateral atelectasis or ground glass appearance
Onion ring fibrosis from a bile duct biopsy should make you think of what diagnosis?	Primary sclerosing cholangitis
What is the minimum amount of time needed for a tick to transfer Lyme disease to a human?	24 hours
What is the most likely diagnosis for a free floating, painless cystic mass found posterior and superior to the testes?	Spermatocele
What heparin complication is relevant to endocrinology?	Adrenal infarct leading to a Cushing's syndrome
What oral antibiotic can be used for pseudomonas?	Ciprofloxacin
What two hormones are secreted by the posterior pituitary?	Oxytocin and antidiuretic hormone (ADH, vasopressin)

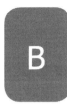

☐	What would you expect to see on a KOH prep if the patient had vaginal candidiasis?	*Pseudohyphae*
☐	Give the definition for preterm labor.	*Contractions that open the cervix before 37 weeks.*
☐	How do you definitively diagnose endometriosis?	*Exploratory laparoscopy*
☐	What is the most common uterine tumor?	*Leiomyoma, also known as fibroids*
☐	What is the most common fracture in children?	*Clavicle*
☐	A fluid filled painless mass found in the scrotum which transilluminates should make you think of what diagnosis?	*Hydrocele*
☐	An HIV patient with ground glass appearance on CXR should make you think of what diagnosis?	*Pneumocystis jiroveci pneumonia (PJP used to be know as PCP)*
☐	Define the third stage of labor.	*Delivery of baby to delivery of placenta.*
☐	What CXR finding might make you think of berylliosis?	*Diffuse infiltrates with hilar adenopathy*
☐	What is the most common type of ovarian cyst?	*Functional cyst - no treatment necessary*
☐	What is the current drug of choice for treating MRSA?	*Vancomycin*
☐	HLA-DR gene is a marker for what endocrine disorder?	*DM type 1*
☐	What is the name for the 4th and 5th metacarpal fractures that often occur punching a wall.	*Boxer's fracture*

B

Tympany to percussion should make you think of what diagonsis?	Large pneuomthorax
What two things are needed to make a diagnosis of bipolar 2?	One major depressive episode and one hypomanic episode.
Gummas or granulomatous nodules should make you think of what diagnosis?	Tertiary syphilis
What are the five components of tetralogy of Fallot?	Ventricular septal defect, right ventricular hypertrophy, right ventricular outflow obstruction (pulmonary valve stenosis), overriding aorta, right sided aortic arch
What is the yellow, brown fleshy mass on the conjunctiva which usually does not interfere with vision?	Pinguecula
Is anorexia egosyntonic or ego-dystonic? What about bulimia?	Anorexia is egosyntonic. Bulimia is ego-dystonic.
At how many weeks of pregnancy can chorionic villus sampling be done?	10-13 weeks
Salmon-colored scales should make you think of what diagnosis?	Psoriasis
Oral herpes is best treated with systemic or topical antivirals?	Topical is the first line. Systemic antivirals will help but are only indicated for severe cases.
What age range is the HPV vaccination recommended for?	9 to 26 years old
What is the more popular term for Stein-Leventhal syndrome.	Polycystic ovarian syndrome

B

☐ What is the most common organism that causes mastitis?	*Staph aureus*
☐ A teardrop lesion after a course of strep throat should make you think of what diagnosis?	*Guttate psoriasis*
☐ When you step up the diagnosis from intermittent asthma to mild persistent asthma what medication should you add?	*An inhaled steroid like fluticasone*
☐ What is the term for a chronic mild depression which has lasted greater than two years?	*Dysthymia*
☐ A patient complains of periumbilical pain which has now moved over McBurney's point. What is the most likely diagnosis?	*Appendicitis*
☐ Which are more painful, hemorrhoids above or below the dentate line?	*Below, internal hemorrhoids are not painful.*
☐ What is it called when a patient says "ee" but on auscultion you here "ay"?	*Egophony*
☐ Stocking glove paresthesias should make you think of what two diagnoses?	*B12 deficiency neuropathy and diabetic neuropathy*
☐ What is the best imaging study for acute appendicitis?	*CT*
☐ What does trismus mean?	*Lock jaw, often secondary to tetanus*
☐ A patient presents with several episodes of vertigo over the past few weeks. He has had intermittent unilateral hearing loss and a "blowing" in his ears. What is the most likely diagnosis?	*Meniere's disease*
☐ A resting or pill-rolling tremor should make you think of what diagnosis?	*Parkinson's disease*

Paradoxical pulses may be found in what pulmonary disorder?	Asthma
Will a patient with achalasia have dysphagia to liquids, solids or both?	Both
An endoscopy for presumed esophagitis shows several solitary deep ulcers. What is the most likely diagnosis?	Cytomegalovirus
What is the #1 cause of small bowel obstruction?	Postoperative adhesions
What is Chvostek's sign?	Tap on facial nerve and get a twitch with low Ca.
What is the most common location for an anal fissure?	Posterior midline
What is the first line antibiotic for otitis media?	Amoxicillin
If you hear crackles in the lung fields list three pulmonary issues that should be in your differential.	Pneumonia, fibrosis, CHF, Bronchitis
What class of medication is first line to treat inflammatory bowel disease in the maintenance phase?	5-ASA products - sulfasalazine, mesalamine
What is the medical term for cross-eyed?	Strabismus
A patient with HIV presents with severe groin pain. What is the most likely diagnosis?	Avascular necrosis of the femoral head. Antiretroviral medications put patients at an increased risk of AVN.
A patient presents with a dense corneal infiltrate and an epithelial defect seen with fluorescein stain. What is the most likely diagnosis?	Corneal ulcer

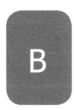

☐	What medication class does metformin (Glucophage) fall into?	*Biguanide*
☐	To be diagnosed with ADD patients must exhibit symptoms before what age?	*7 years old*
☐	What is the heart rate for tachycardia? How about bradycardia?	*Tachycardia >100, bradycardia <60*
☐	What is the least aggressive thyroid cancer?	*Papillary*
☐	At what age should vaccinations for pneumococcal pneumonia begin?	*65 years old*
☐	Which is the most commonly herniated vertebral disc?	*L4-L5 followed by L5-S1*
☐	When is the typical onset of Tourette's syndrome?	*3-8 years old*
☐	Will unconjugated bilirubin be high or low in a patient with sickle cell disease?	*High*
☐	What is the most serious complication of Kawasaki syndrome?	*Aortic Aneurysm*
☐	List three class 1a antiarrhythmics.	*Disopyramide, quinidine, procainamide*
☐	What are the four muscles of the rotator cuff?	*Commonly referred to as the SITS muscles they are Supraspinatus, Infraspinatus, Teres minor, Subscapularis*
☐	How do you treat hookworm?	*Azoles*
☐	What is the most common cause of lower GI bleed?	*Diverticulosis*

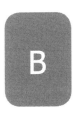

☐ Typically what is the first medication started in type 2 DM?	*Metformin*
☐ You hear a loud harsh holosystolic murmur in a child. It is heard best at the LLSB. What diagnosis should you be thinking of?	*Ventricular septal defect*
☐ A positive Neer's test indicates what diagnosis?	*Rotator cuff impingement*
☐ A pearly dome-shaped lesion with a central umbilication should make you think of what diagnosis?	*Molluscum contagiousum*
☐ Antisocial personality disorder may not be diagnosed until what age?	*18 years old*
☐ What is the most common patient complaint with emphysema?	*Shortness of breath*
☐ List the components of Virchow's triad.	*Stasis, vascular injury, hypercoagulability*
☐ Give two classes of drug therapy for treating parkinson's.	*Dopaminergic (levodopa), anticholinergics are second line*
☐ Asplenism secondary to sickle cell disease increases a patient's risk for what type of infections?	*Capsulated organisms like Strep pneumo and H. flu.*
☐ Which carpal bone has a high rate of nonunion and occult fracture?	*Scaphoid*
☐ What is the defining symptom of Alzheimer's?	*Progressive memory impairment*
☐ A patient presents with knee pain following a soccer game two days ago. He has joint line tenderness medially and feels a locking in the knee from time to time. What two physical exam tests should you do?	*This is probably a medial meniscal tear. McMurry and apply tests would be appropriate.*

B

- [ ] What might you feel on a digital rectal exam of a patient with prostate cancer?

  Enlarged prostate, hard nodules within the prostate

- [ ] What is the most common cause of DM type 1?

  Autoimmune destruction of the islet cells in the pancreas

- [ ] What is the drug of choice for toxoplasmosis?

  Bactrim

- [ ] What is the age range for osteosarcoma? Where are they most typically found in the body?

  Osteosarcoma usually occur in 15-25 year old males and are most commonly found around the knee.

- [ ] What does HBsAg (hep B surface antigen) indicate?

  Active Hep B infection

- [ ] White oral lesions which can be scraped off leaving punctate bleeding should make you think of what diagnosis?

  Oral candida

- [ ] Pregnant woman and cat litter should make you think of what diagnosis?

  Toxoplasmosis

- [ ] What is necessary to diagnose a patient with bipolar 1?

  One manic episode. They do not have to have the depressive episode for the diagnosis.

- [ ] What are the two main causes of aortic stenosis?

  Congenital bicuspid valve and calcification of the valve secondary to coronary artery disease

- [ ] Are hallucinations normal during a normal grieving period?

  Yes, as long as they are not persistent or intrusive.

- [ ] Is the ankle jerk reflex of lumbar or sacral origin?

  Sacral

- [ ] How do you treat an H. pylori infection?

  PPI + 2 antibiotics, commonly omeprazole + clarithromycin and amoxicillin or PPI + metronidazole + tetracycline

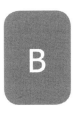

What area of the prostate is the primary site for prostate cancer?	The peripheral zone
What is the most common preceding event for orbital cellulitis?	URI
What organism causes toxoplasmosis?	*Toxoplasma gondii*
A thumbprint sign on an abdominal film should make you think of what diagnosis?	Intestinal ischemia
In what age range do you expect to most commonly find amaurosis fugax?	Patients older than 50
Is glaucoma more prevalent in males or females?	Females 3:1
What is the initial treatment for a myocardial infarction?	MONA - morphine, oxygen, nitroglycerin and aspirin
What medication is clearly contraindicated in anorexia and bulimia?	Bupropion (Wellbutrin) because it can increase risk of seizures.
Rhonchi or wheezes that clear after coughing suggest what diagnosis?	Bronchitis or atelectasis
Maltese crosses in the urine should make you think of what diagnosis?	Nephrotic syndrome
What imaging needs to be done before taking a patient to the OR with an aortic aneurysm?	CT (echo may be used as initial study, but CT is need for surgery)
What three labs should you order if you are considering secondary amenorrhea?	beta-HCG, TSH, Prolactin
What is first line treatment for rosacea?	Metronidazole, tetracycline is probably a close second.

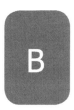

- You are counting boxes from the peak of a QRS wave on an EKG in order to determine the heart rate. What would the heart rate be if the next QRS wave peak were three boxes away? What numbers are associated with the first five boxes?

    The answer is 100. The heart rates by conting boxes are 300, 150, 100, 75, 60.

- What are three causes for a postpartum hemorrhage?

    Uterine atony, genital laceration, retained placenta

- A 65 year old presents complaining of severe pain in his great toe that began when he woke up this morning. It is swollen, red and very tender. What is the most likely diagnosis?

    Gout would be number one because of the location, but you might also think about an infection.

- An involuntary loss of urine during coughing or laughing is what type of incontinence?

    Stress incontinence

- What is the management of a patient in supraventricular tachycardia?

    Vagal maneuvers, carotid massage, adenosine

- What is the clinical name for whooping cough?

    Pertussis

- A patient is having a stroke and there is no evidence of hemorrhage. What is the first line medical treatment?

    Within the first 4 hours and with no contraindications thrombolytics should be given.

- What is the generic name for Prozac?

    Fluoxetine

- List three things that should be in your differential if you hear wheezes on a lung exam?

    Asthma, COPD, Bronchitis

- Thin, sticky, malodorous vaginal discharge should make you think of what diagnosis?

    Bacterial vaginosis

- What percentage of strokes are ischemic? What percentage are hemorrhagic?

    80%, 20%

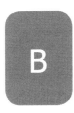

☐ Koplik spots are white clustered lesions on the buccal mucosa. What virus are they pathognomonic for?	*Measles/Rubeola*
☐ List two common offending agents for pill induced esophagitis?	*NSAIDS, KCl, iron, antibiotics*
☐ Currant jelly sputum should make you think of what diagnosis?	*Klebsiella pneumoniae*
☐ A Gram-negative diplococci should make you think of what diagnosis?	*Neisseria*
☐ What are three medications often combined as a first line treatment for H. pylori?	*Omeprazole, clarithromycin and amoxicillin (PPI + 2 Antibioitcs)*
☐ When does quickening occur?	*Nulliparous 18-20 weeks, multiparous 14-16 weeks*
☐ Clue cells should make you think of what diagnosis?	*Bacterial vaginosis*
☐ What tumor marker may be used for liver cancer?	*alpha-Fetoprotein*
☐ Which NSAID has the highest rate of peptic ulceration?	*Naproxen*
☐ What is the mean age for ovarian cancer?	*63, you will need to think of this in an older patient with vague abdominal symptoms.*
☐ Define threatened abortion.	*Vaginal bleeding, closed cervix, products of conception are still inside*
☐ A patient presents with a painful, red nodule on the eyelid. What is the most likely diagnosis? What treatment should you begin with?	*Hordeolum (sty). Warm compress and progress to topical antibiotics if necessary.*
☐ You notice a bowing of the iris on exam. What diagnosis should you be thinking of?	*Glaucoma*

B

☐	Are most shoulder dislocations anterior or posterior?	Anterior
☐	Where is disease of the pulmonary valve best heard?	2nd left intercostal space
☐	What is the definitive treatment for cardiac tamponade?	Pericardiocentesis
☐	A patient has pneumonia with rust colored sputum. What is the most likely diagnosis?	Strep pneumonia
☐	A blockage of which artery causes an anterior wall MI?	Left anterior descending artery
☐	List four indications for the flu vaccine.	Child 6-59 months, pregnant female, healthcare worker, age greater than 50
☐	A CXR shows a "3" sign with notching of the ribs. What is the most likely diagnosis?	Coarctation of the aorta
☐	List four diagnostic criteria for diabetes?	Random glucose >200, fasting glucose >126, two hour postprandial glucose >200, HgA1c >6.5%
☐	A patient has a GFR of 25 and HTN. Which class should you use, a loop or a thiazide diuretic?	A loop will work no matter how low the GFR is. Thiazides will only work with a GFR over 30.
☐	Describe the characteristics of a lytic lesion on x-ray.	Spiculated, elevated periosteum, bone destruction (think bad, very bad things)
☐	List three possible treatments for stress incontinence in women.	Kegels, estrogen therapy, surgical placement of a urethral sling
☐	How does levothyroxine work?	It is a synthetic T4

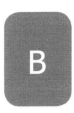

☐ You are treating a patient for TB. He has noticed that his body fluids now have an orange tint. What drug is most likely causing this?	*Rifampin*
☐ List 4 risk factors for endometrial cancer.	*Chronic unopposed estrogen, nulliparity, early menarche, late menopause, tamoxifen, DM, obesity, HTN, breast cancer, ovarian cancer*
☐ Where is the epididymis found?	*It is found at the posterior upper pole.*
☐ A patient with a history of asthma presents complaining of stringy discharge from both eyes and severe swelling around the eyes. What is the most likely diagnosis?	*Allergic conjunctivitis*
☐ What are the most common primary cancer sites for metastasis to the brain?	*Lung, breast, kidney*
☐ What type of hearing loss is associated with aging?	*Sensory*
☐ What type of organism causes botulism?	*A Gram + rod, Clostridium botulinum*
☐ What is the first line medical treatment for stage 1 hypertension?	*Thiazide diuretic*
☐ Honey-colored crusts should make you think of what diagnosis?	*Impetigo*
☐ Fasting gastrin will be above what level with gastrinoma?	*>150 pg/ml*
☐ What is the main risk factor for esophagitis?	*Immunocompromised patient*
☐ Most gallstones are made of what substance?	*Cholesterol*
☐ List 4 physical exam findings for Cushing's syndrome.	*Moon face, buffalo hump, purple striae, central obesity, supraclavicular fat pads, easy bruising*

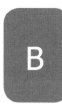

☐	Bruises may be purple, green, yellow and brown. How many days old is a yellow bruise?	*Purple day 1-5, Green day 5-7, Yellow 7-10, Brown 10-14*
☐	An 18 month old is not yet speaking. He does not point to objects. He does not make eye contact with others. What diagnosis should you be thinking of?	*Autism*
☐	How does metformin work?	*Decreases the hepatic glucose production and increases peripheral glucose uptake.*
☐	An endoscopy for presumed esophagitis shows multiple shallow ulcers. What is the most likely diagnosis?	*Herpes simplex virus*
☐	What is the single most important thing to be concerned about with a patient in status epilepticus?	*Airway, followed by management of hyperthermia.*
☐	Hyperinflation on a CXR as well as eosinophilia on CBC should make you think of what diagnosis?	*Asthma*
☐	What is the most common endometrial cancer?	*75% are adenocarcinomas*
☐	Is surgery curative for Crohn's or ulcerative colitis?	*Ulcerative colitis*
☐	What class of antibiotics should you start with for community acquired pneumonia?	*Macrolides*
☐	A patient presents with a painless mass in her right wrist. What is the most likely diagnosis?	*Ganglion cyst*
☐	How do you treat polymyalgia rheumatica?	*Low dose prednisone*
☐	A patient presents to the ER with acute progessive weakness, diplopia and a very dry mouth. What organism may be causing this?	*Clostridium botulinum*

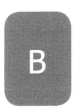

☐	A 3 year old boy presents with hematuria and a painless palpable abdominal mass. What diagnosis should you be thinking of?	Wilms tumor
☐	What is the diagnostic test of choice for Zenker's diverticulum?	Barium swallow will show the diverticulum.
☐	The term satellite lesion should make you think of what diagnosis?	Candida diaper rash
☐	What is the most common cause of pneumonia in children less than 1 year old?	Respiratory syncytial virus (RSV)
☐	What is the medical treatment for an early ectopic pregnancy?	Methotrexate
☐	Alcohol may be a major factor in which encephalopathy?	Wernicke's
☐	Hyperresonance to percussion should make you think of what diagonsis?	Emphysema, pneumothorax, asthma
☐	A sponge-like prostate on digital rectal exam should make you think of what diagnosis?	Prostatitis, but be careful. You can cause sepsis with a digital rectal exam.
☐	A 45 year old female complains of feeling the ground rolling under her feet at times. What is the most likely diagnosis?	Vertigo
☐	List three medications used to "treat" multiple sclerosis?	Steroids, interferon beta, copolymer 1
☐	A patient with primary amenorrhea and a low FSH should make you think of what diagnosis?	Hypothalamic pituitary insufficiency
☐	A kidney stone of less than what size will likely pass on its own?	Less than 5 mm
☐	What are the two most common organisms responsible for cellulitis?	Strep and Staph

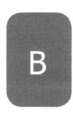

☐ Define incomplete abortion.	*Vaginal bleeding, cervix is open, products of conception partially passed*
☐ What is the most useful physical exam test for diagnosing an ACL tear?	*Lachman's, followed by anterior drawer*
☐ What is the drug of choice for the treatment of Lyme disease?	*Doxycicline*
☐ A patient complains of severe pleuritic chest pain that is relieved with sitting and leaning forward. What is the most likely diagnosis?	*Pericarditis*
☐ List two diagnoses which require antibiotic prophylaxis for "dirty procedures?"	*Prosthetic valve, valve repair with any prosthetic material, prior endocarditis diagnosis, congenital cyanotic heart defect*
☐ List two risk factors for prostate cancer.	*Advancing age, African American, positive family history, high fat diet*
☐ What three symptoms are classic for a normal pressure hydrocephalus?	*Gait disturbance, dementia and urinary incontinence*
☐ Which thyroid cancer is the most aggressive?	*Anaplastic*
☐ What antibiotic is most likely to cause C. diff?	*Clindamycin*
☐ You think a patient may have an osteoid osteoma due to his complaints of severe night pain. You set him up for an x-ray; but in the meantime what medication do you start him on?	*If it is truly an osteoid osteoma ibuprofen will resolve his pain.*
☐ Why should actinic keratosis be treated?	*It may progress to squamous cell carcinoma.*

B

A patient presents with unproductive retching, acute localized epigastric distention and inability to pass a nasogastric tube. What is the most likely diagnosis?	Gastric volvulus
Pretibial myxedema should make you think of what diagnosis?	Graves' disease
Is Huntington's autosomal dominant or recessive?	Dominant
What medication is used for patients with lupus?	Systemic steroids
Moans, groans, stones and bones describe symptoms of what endocrine problem?	Hyperparathyroid
What is erythema nodosum?	Tender red nodules usually found on the shins.
Dullness to percussion should make you think of what diagonsis?	Lobar pneumonia
A snowstorm appearance on ultrasound should make you think of what diagnosis?	Hydatidiform mole
What is the first line medical treatment for a patient who presents with palpitations and nervousness secondary to hyperthyroidism?	Beta Blockers
Which EKG leads are used to diagnose an anterolateral MI?	V5 and V6
What is a common symptom that goes along with chest pain for GERD patients?	Dry cough
When treating psychiatric patients are benzodiazepines used more commonly for acute or chronic treatment?	Acute
What medium do you need to grow out Neisseria gonorrhoeae?	Thayer-Martin

B

Hyperpigmentation of the skin along creases should make you think of what diagnosis?	Addison's disease
Mesothelioma is most commonly found in what lung location?	80% are found in the pleural lining.
The description of a dew drop on a rose petal should make you think of what diagnosis?	Chickenpox
What is the first line treatment for pertussis?	Erythromycin
How do you administer the Weber hearing test?	Tuning fork placed in the middle of the forehead.
What medication used in hepatitis B infection helps prevent the need for liver transplant?	Lamivudine
An x-ray of the skull reveals coalescence of mastoid air cells. What is the most likely diagnosis?	Mastoiditis
How long should you wait for a swallowed marble to pass through the body before considering surgery?	24 hours
You should be thinking alpha thalassemia if the question stem includes which four geographic areas?	Southeast Asia, China, Middle East, Africa
How do you treat pneumocystis jiroveci pneumonia (PCJ) formerly known as pneumocystis pneumonia (PCP)?	Bactrim
Bullae and blebs on CXR should make you think of what diagnosis?	Emphysema
How do you define 1st degree AV block?	The PR interval is longer than 0.2 seconds or one block on EKG.

B

An African American teenager presents with avascular necrosis of the his right femoral head. What diagnosis should you be thinking of?	*Sickle cell disease*
A patient presents with what appears to be an inability to understand speech. Which aphasia should be at the top of your differential?	*Wernicke's aphasia*
By what age should a child be able to kick a ball?	*24 months*
What is the most common cause of hypoparathyroid?	*Post thyroidectomy with the complication of parathyroidectomy.*
How many days after conception is a serum beta-HCG positive?	*8*
What is the name of the test for dry eyes?	*Schirmer's test*
You have a patient with PCOS who would like to get pregnant. What are two medications you may start her on?	*Metformin and Clomid*
What is the term for painful swallowing?	*Odynophagia*
Which hyperlipidemia medication may cause flushing?	*Niacin*
List three risk factors for an ectopic pregnancy.	*Previous ectopic, scarred tubes (hx of PID or salpingitis), IUD*
How do statins work to affect the lipid profile?	*They slow the rate limiting step of cholesterol synthesis*
How often should patients with pernicious anemia have a screening endoscopy performed?	*Every 5 years looking for signs of gastric carcinoma*
A patient presents with irregular menses, hirsutism and infertility. What is the most likely diagnosis?	*Polycystic ovarian syndrome*

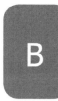

☐	If you have heartburn that does not improve with medication what diagnosis should you be thinking about?	*Gastrinoma*
☐	What siezure medication may cause overgrowth of the gums?	*Phenytoin*
☐	What medical treatment is given for a gastrinoma?	*Proton pump inhibitors*
☐	You suspect a patient has polyarteritis nodosa. What is the test for a definitive diagnosis and what is the treatment?	*Biopsy, high dose steroids*
☐	How do you treat pityriasis rosea?	*Reassurance*
☐	In a folic acid deficiency anemia the folic acid level is typically below what level?	*<150*
☐	What is the treatment for a volvulus in a child?	*Barium enema*
☐	Which is associated with painful third trimester bleeding placental abruption or placenta previa?	*Placental abruption*
☐	What would you expect the WBC count to be in the joint fluid of an infected knee?	*>50,000 at a minimum and probably much higher*
☐	What are three treatments for uterine prolapse?	*Pessary, Kegel's maneuvers, surgical repair*
☐	What type of hallucinations are most common in schizophrenia auditory, visual or olfactory?	*Auditory - hearing voices*
☐	A very sick patient with diffuse infiltrates that spare the costophrenic angles should make you think of what diagnosis?	*Acute respiratory distress syndrome (ARDS)*
☐	Severe abdominal pain 30 minutes after a meal should make you think of what diagnosis?	*Intestinal ischemia*

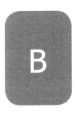

A widely split fixed S2 should make you think of what diagnosis?	Atrial septal defect
Diabetes insipidus is caused by a deficiency of which hormone?	Vasopressin
What is the best test for diagnosing Rocky Mountain spotted fever?	Indirect immunofluorescent antibodies
Left lower quadrant pain and tenderness should make you think of what diagnosis?	Diverticulitis
A patient with mitral valve prolapse will often have what physical characteristics?	Often a thin female
What is the name of the sign when a patient shows inhibited inspiration with pressure over the RUQ? What diagnosis does it suggest?	Murphy's sign, Cholecystitis
A unilateral, single, mobile, firm, nontender solid breast mass should make you think of what diagnosis?	Fibroadenoma
Tenderness at the costovertebral angle should make you think of what diagnosis?	Pyelonephritis
Who is more likely to have an aortic aneurysm males or females?	Males are eight times as likely to have an aortic aneurysm.
An ABG shows a pH of 7.2, a bicarb of 25 and a PCO2 of 50. Is this respiratory or metabolic acidosis?	Respiratory - CO2 is elevated
Define the second stage of labor.	Fully dilated to delivery
What medication might you use prior to a thyroidectomy in a patient with hyperthyroidism?	Methimazole or propylthiouracil (PTU)

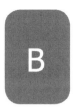

☐ A patient presents complaining of the worst headache of his life. What might you expect their blood pressure to be?	*Typically this is the description for a subarachnoid hemorrhage. You would expect the blood pressure to be elevated.*
☐ Syphilis is caused by what organism?	*Treponema pallidum*
☐ A sudden thunderclap headache should make you think of what diagnosis?	*Subarachnoid hematoma*
☐ How do you treat a stasis dermatitis?	*Compression stockings*
☐ What class of cardiac medications should be avoided in patients with asthma?	*Beta blockers (blocks receptors for bronchodilators)*
☐ A patient presents with a hot potato or muffled voice. What is the most likely diagnosis?	*Peritonsillar abscess*
☐ What is the term for being afraid of being out in a terrible situation with no help available?	*Agoraphobia*
☐ At what age should a child begin to say momma and dadda?	*12 months*
☐ What is the imaging study of choice if you suspect bladder cancer?	*Cystoscopy and biopsy*
☐ How do you treat alcohol withdrawal?	*Benzodiazepines*
☐ The heart rate is irregular, so you can't count boxes between QRS waves to determine heart rate. What is another method you can use to determine rate on an EKG?	*Count QRS waves in a six second strip and multiply by 10 to get beats per minute.*
☐ What is the term for bilateral yellow plaques near the eyes?	*Xanthelasma*
☐ What is the first line treatment for genital warts?	*Imiquimod (Aldara)*

B

What organism has been linked to reactive arthritis?	*Shigella, also remember that reactive arthritis has a positive HLA-B27.*
What is the most common cause of postrenal renal failure?	*BPH, postrenal renal failure is secondary to an outflow obstruction*
A patient complains of a rash on his palms and soles. He has a fever and chills. In conversation he mentions a strange painless chancre he had a few weeks ago. What diagnosis should you be thinking of?	*Secondary syphilis. This is the most contagious stage.*
A patient is bitten by a rabies infected raccoon. On what days do you give human diploid cells?	*0,3,7,14,28*
What is pica?	*Eating non-food items including ice, paper, dirt, hair*
Pale and boggy nasal mucosa should make you think of what diagnosis?	*Allergic rhinitis*
If the pap smear results come back anything other than negative or ASCUS what is your next step?	*Colposcopy and biopsy*
Rheumatic fever most commonly affects which valve?	*The mitral valve*
Name one aldosterone antagonist.	*Spironolactone, eplerenone*
Currant jelly stool should make you think of what diagnosis?	*Intussusception*
What is the normal range of fetal heart rate?	*120-160*
How long before normal grief resolves?	*About one year*
The accessory pathway known as the James bundle should make you think of what syndrome?	*Lown-Ganong-Levine syndrome*

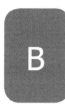

☐	What does Anti-HBs (hep B surface antibody) indicate?	*Recovery from infection or immunization to hepatitis B*
☐	Steatorrhea should make you think of what diagnosis?	*Pancreatitis*
☐	An EEG showing generalized spikes and associated slow waves should make you think of what diagnosis?	*Generalized or absence seizure*
☐	Does adenocarcinoma arise from the proximal or distal esophagus?	*Distal*
☐	What is Hashimoto's disease?	*An autoimmune cause of hypothyroid.*
☐	How much time needs to pass before diagnosing secondary amenorrhea?	*If cycles have been normal 3 months. If cycles have been irregular 6 months.*
☐	What is the best treatment for molluscum contagiosum?	*It is self limiting, but can be removed if patient really wants it.*
☐	A patient presents with facial paresis, arm drift and abnormal speech. What are the first three tests to order?	*Thinking of a stroke you order a non-contrast brain CT or MRI, serum glucose and oxygen saturation.*
☐	What is the treatment for Addison's disease?	*Hydrocortisone or prednisone*
☐	What age range is typically associated with testicular torsion?	*10-20 years old*
☐	Will serum potassium be decreased or elevated in renal failure?	*Elevated*
☐	A patient complains of regurgitating undigested food several hours after a meal. What diagnosis should you be thinking of?	*Zenker's diverticulum*
☐	Fruity breath should make you think of what diagnosis?	*Diabetic ketoacidosis*

B

A fundal exam shows an opalescent retina and boxcarring of arterioles. What diagnosis should you be thinking of?	Central retinal artery occlusion
Caseating granulomas should make you think of what diagnosis?	TB
A double comedone is indicative of what diagnosis?	Hidradenitis suppurativa
A pathologic S3 is most commonly associated with what diagnosis?	CHF
What is Tietze syndrome?	Costochondritis
An HIV patient presents with a nonproductive cough and a CXR showing diffuse interstitial infiltrates. What diagnosis should you be thinking of?	Pneumocystis jiroveci pneumonia (PCJ) formerly known as Pneumocystis pneumonia (PCP)
What is the most common cause of a hip dislocation? Is it usually anterior or posterior?	MVA, posterior
What is the most common anorectal problem affecting patients over 50?	Hemorrhoids
A herald patch should make you think of what diagnosis?	Pityriasis rosea
List one major risk factor for bladder cancer?	Smoking
How do you treat lichen simplex chronicus?	Get the patient to stop scratching it.
A 14 year old field hockey player presents with prominent adenopathy, white purple exudates in the throat and a palpable spleen. What is the most likely diagnosis?	Mononucleosis
Cortical adrenal insufficiency is also known as what disease?	Addison's disease

What is a good beta blocker to reduce portal HTN?	*Propranolol*
An exudative pleural effusion should make you think of what diagnosis?	*TB, Lung cancer and pneumonia*
On physical exam, you hear a harsh systolic murmur along the right sternal border. What is the most likely diagnosis?	*Aortic stenosis*
List the three diagnosis you should be thinking of if a question includes Heinz bodies.	*G6PD deficiency anemia, chronic liver disease, alpha thalassemia*
What is the best imaging for a thyroid nodule?	*Ultrasound*
What disease is defined as an immunologic response to gluten?	*Celiac*
A patient complains of acute paralysis in his left arm. This does not seem to bother him, but his wife made him come in. There was no traumatic event. A complete neurologic workup is negative. What diagnosis should you be thinking of?	*Conversion disorder*
Purulent cervical discharge should make you think of what diagnosis?	*Neisseria gonorrhoeae*
What is the most common cause of dementia?	*Alzheimer's disease, it may be as high as 80%.*
Are lesions from psoriasis typically found on flexor or extensor surfaces?	*Extensor*
What is the most likely diagnosis for a young man who experiences sudden death while playing sports?	*Hypertrophic cardiomyopathy*
Rice water stool should make you think of what diagnosis?	*Cholera*

B

☐	At what size induration would a PPD be positive for an HIV patient?	5mm
☐	Crohn's is found where in the GI tract?	It can be from esophagus to anus.
☐	What is the age range for Duchenne's muscular dystrophy?	3-5 years old
☐	What is the normal range for MCV?	80-100
☐	A colonoscopy that shows cobblestone or skip lesions should make you think of what diagnosis?	Crohn's disease
☐	What is the most common congenital heart defect?	Ventricular septal defect
☐	What two viral hepatitis infections are self limiting?	Hepatitis A and hepatitis E
☐	What role does C-peptide play in the diagnosis of diabetes?	It is a marker of insulin production. Elevated C-peptide points to DM 2. Decreased C-peptide points towards DM 1.
☐	A patient believes that her 15 year old daughter is sleeping with the mailman. She has no evidence of this. She has confronted her daughter who denies it. It is not interfering with her daily activities, but she does spend time thinking about it. What diagnosis should you be thinking of?	Delusional disorder
☐	What is the gold standard for the diagnosis of cystic fibrosis?	Sweat chloride test
☐	What is the term for an abscess in the sacrococcygeal cleft?	Pilonidal disease
☐	How do you treat bacterial vaginosis?	Metronidazole x 7 days
☐	Which lipid medication may cause flushing?	Niacin

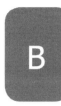

☐	List the three most commonly used medical treatments for COPD?	*Oxygen, ipratropium and albuterol*
☐	What are the main side effects of isoniazid?	*Hepatitis and peripheral neuropathy*
☐	Muddy-brown sediment in the urine should make you think of what diagnosis?	*Acute tubular necrosis*
☐	Are target cells seen in mild or severe iron deficiency anemia?	*Severe, they are also seen in alpha thalassemia, chronic liver disease and asplenia.*
☐	What are the five components of the biophysical profile as part of antepartum testing?	*A non-stress test, fetal breathing, two gross body movements, fetal tone, amniotic fluid index*
☐	Should a breast feeding mother stop breast feeding if she develops mastitis?	*Mastitis is not in itself a reason to stop breast feeding. An abcess would be an a indication to stop.*
☐	Community acquired carditis is most often caused by one of the HACEK organisms. List the HACEK organisms.	*Haemophilus, Actinobacillus, Cardiobacterium, Eikenella, Kingella*
☐	What is the most accurate way to diagnose urethritis?	*Urine PCR*
☐	What is the name of the syndrome that involves pericarditis several days after a myocardial infarction?	*Dressler syndrome*
☐	What is the most common cause of secondary hypertension?	*Chronic kidney disease*
☐	Define orthostatic hypotension.	*A drop in systolic blood pressure of >20 mmhg when standing up.*
☐	A patient has just received a cardiac stent. How long will he be on aspirin and clopidogrel?	*One year*

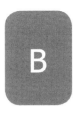

What might happen if you infuse vancomycin too fast?	Red Man syndrome
What two lung cancers are typically found peripherally on CXR?	Adenocarcinoma and Large cell
A child with a fever lasting longer than five days should make you think of what diagnosis?	Kawasaki syndrome
Tall peaked P waves should make you think of what diagnosis?	Right atrial enlargement
Grape-like vesicles or a sack of grapes on ultrasound should make you think of what diagnosis?	Hydatidiform mole
What medication might you switch to if a patient develops an intolerable cough on an ACEI?	Angiotensin receptor blocker (ARBs)
In a patient with hyperthyroidism will TSH most likely be elevated or decreased?	Decreased
How is acute stress disorder different than posttraumatic stress disorder?	Acute stress disorder occurs within 1 month of event and resolves within about a month. PTSD begins at about 1 month after event and can last indefinitely.
By what age should a child be able to roll over?	4 months
List the five major Jones criteria for diagnosing rheumatic fever.	Polyarthritis, carditis, subcuticular nodes, erythema marginatum, chorea
G6PD deficiency follows what pattern of inheritance?	X-linked

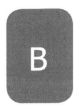

☐ A 65 year old male presents with frequency. On digital rectal exam you feel an elastic moderately enlarged prostate. What diagnosis should you be thinking of?	BPH
☐ What is the first line treatment for orbital cellulitis?	IV antibiotics, followed by 2 weeks of oral antibiotics.
☐ An opening snap on auscultation of the heart should make you think of what diagnosis?	Mitral stenosis
☐ A continuous murmur most likely involves what area of the heart?	It is most likely a septal defect
☐ A patient believes she is pregnant. You notice that her cervix appears a little blue. What is the name of this sign?	Chadwick's sign
☐ Pizza pie retinopathy should make you think of what diagnosis?	Cytomegalovirus (CMV)
☐ Postmenopausal bleeding is immediately believed to be what diagnosis?	Endometrial cancer until proven otherwise.
☐ A young child presents to ER and you see him waiting in tripod position. What is the most likely diagnosis?	Epiglottitis
☐ List two medications commonly used for hypertension in pregnancy.	Methyldopa and labetalol
☐ What is the first line medical treatment for torsades de pointes?	Magnesium sulfate
☐ List three drugs that treat cluster headaches.	Oxygen, sumatriptan, butorphanol
☐ What is the first line treatment for a varicocele?	Watchful waiting unless there is a question of fertility.

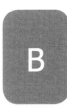

What hematological disorder should you think of if the questions talks about the patient eating ice or dirt?	*Iron deficiency anemia*
What is the current drug of choice for the cytomegalovirus?	*Ganciclovir*
If you see a question with anything to do with rats and the patient has pneumonia, what organism should you be thinking of?	*Yersinia pestis*
A Salter-Harris type I fracture affects what area of the bone?	*Only the physis (growth plate)*
As it relates to diabetics, what is the dawn phenomenon?	*Reduced insulin response between 5 and 8 am*
List the four things that suggest group A beta-hemolytic strep in a patient with pharyngitis.	*Fever, tender anterior cervical adenopathy, no cough and an exudate in the throat*
You have a patient with pulsus paradoxus. What two diagnosis should you be thinking of?	*Cardiac tamponade, pericarditis and pulmonary obstructive lung diseases (think COPD)*
Inability to absorb vitamin B12 due to lack of intrinsic factor is what disease?	*Pernicious anemia*
What is the most common cause of secondary amenorrhea?	*Pregnancy*
What ejection fraction is typical for a patient with CHF?	*35-40%*
After a thiazide diuretic, what medication should you start in a hypertensive patient who also has diabetes?	*An ACEI or an ARB*

B

When treating herpes keratitis should you use topical antivirals, topical steroids or both?	Don't use steroids. Topical antiviral and refer!
An elevated serum amylase and lipase should make you think of what diagnosis?	Pancreatitis
A pearl formation on CXR should make you think of what diagnosis?	Squamous cell lung cancer
Will epididymitis feel better with scrotal elevation?	Yes
Define priapism.	Painful persistent erection
A patient has metamorphopsia and a central blind spot. What is the most likely diagnosis?	Macular degeneration
What is the drug of choice to treat a urethritis caused by neisseria?	Ceftriaxone (Rocephin)
A CT scan shows ring enhancing lesions in an HIV patient. What diagnosis should you be thinking of?	Toxoplasmosis
What is the treatment for botulism?	Antitoxin
Silvery scales should make you think of what diagnosis?	Psoriasis
Which is more likely to pass into the scrotum, a direct or indirect hernia?	Indirect
A dendritic lesion is seen with fluorescein stain. What is the most likely diagnosis?	Herpes keratitis
Are fibrocystic breast masses usually bilateral or unilateral?	Bilateral
What two antibiotics are used for empiric treatment of endocarditis?	Vancomycin and ceftriaxone together are first line empiric treatment.

B

When is it recommended to begin pap smears?	New guidlines suggest to begin testing women at age 21 and not before.
A patient complains of seeing halos and rainbows around lights. She also complains of moderate photophobia? What is the most likely diagnosis?	Glaucoma
Pica is often related to what type of anemia?	Iron deficiency anemia
What are three things in your differential if you have a paradoxical pulse?	Cardiac tamponade, pericarditis and pulmonary obstructive lung diseases (think COPD)
In a patient with sensorineural hearing loss, what will be the results of the Weber test?	The patient will hear the sound louder in the unaffected ear.
What is the most common cause of a folate deficiency?	Alcoholism
With a gastric ulcer are the patient's symptoms exacerbated or relieved with food?	Exacerbated
Both lead I and AVF have positive QRS complexes. Does this represent normal axis, left axis deviation or right axis deviation?	Normal axis
What endocrine issue is associated with PCOS?	Insulin insensitivity
Large doughy hands should make you think of what diagnosis?	Gigantism
Early on in pregnancy serial beta-HCG should double over what time period?	every 48-72 hours
At what age and how often should fecal occult blood tests be performed as a screening tool?	Beginning at age 50, and they should be done every year.
What virus causes mumps?	Paramyxovirus

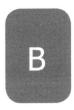

☐	Strict vegans are at risk for what type of anemia?	B12 deficiency anemia
☐	Which lab should be tightly monitored in a patient taking an aldosterone antagonist?	Potassium, they may have hyperkalemia
☐	At what size induration would a PPD be positive for a healthcare worker?	10mm
☐	Oval patches of hair loss should make you think of what diagnosis?	Alopecia areata
☐	What is the most common pituitary adenoma?	Prolactinoma
☐	List two ectopic tumors that may produce ACTH and give a patient Cushing's syndrome?	Small cell lung cancer, pancreatic islet cells, thymomas
☐	Define missed abortion.	No vaginal bleeding, cervix is closed, products of conception are still inside
☐	What type of behavioral therapy works best for borderline patients?	Dialectical behavior therapy
☐	The pap smear results on a 23 year old patient come back as atypical squamous cell uncertain significance (ASCUS). What is your next step?	Repeat pap smear in 12 months although HPV test is acceptable.
☐	Extremely pruritic lesions with burrows in runs should make you think of what diagnosis?	Scabies
☐	Which is the most commonly affected sinus in acute sinusitis?	Maxillary
☐	What two valvular issues do patients with Marfan's syndrome often have?	Aortic regurgitation and mitral valve prolapse (you can tell them apart by where they are heard).
☐	A cervical biopsy comes back as CIN2 or CIN3. What is your next step?	Excision - LEEP, Cold knife (worry about incompetent cervix), Cryotherapy

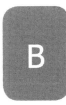

How do you treat allergic rhinitis?	Intranasal corticosteroid and antihistamines
A positive Auspitz sign should make you think of what diagnosis?	Psoriasis
A patient complains of muscle weakness and fatigability that improves with rest. What diagnosis should you be thinking of?	Myasthenia gravis
What is represented by ST segment depressions greater than 1mm on EKG?	Ischemia
A patient in the ER has no pulse; but on EKG, there are wide irregular "complexes" which are at an irregular rate. They all appear very different from one another. What is the treatment for this patient?	He is in ventricular fibrillation. The treatment is defibrillation.
What is the appropriate treatment for central vein occlusion?	Typically self limited. Treat underlying disease.
A patient with a history of herpes now presents with a target lesion. What is the most likely diagnosis?	Erythema multiforme
A patient with a history of smoking presents with a new onset hoarseness. This has been persistant for the past two weeks. What is the most likely diagnosis?	Laryngeal squamous cell carcinoma
A fundal exam shows a cup to disc ratio of >0.5. There are also vessels bending over the disc. What is the most likely diagnosis?	Glaucoma
List the four most common places lung cancer will metastasize to?	Bone, brain, adrenals and liver
A patient has a history of multiple stys. He now has a painless nodule on his eyelid and minor conjunctivitis. What is the most likely diagnosis?	Chalazion

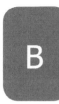

☐ What are the two most common predisposing factors in the development of chronic renal failure?	HTN and DM
☐ List three catastrophic complications of a myocardial infarction.	Papillary muscle rupture, myocardial wall rupture and left ventricular aneurysm
☐ Is staph gram (+) or gram (−)?	Gram (+)
☐ What is the other term for Mobitz type I?	Wenckebach
☐ Do loop diuretics cause hyperkalemia or hypokalemia?	Hypokalemia
☐ Is obsessive compulsive disorder egosyntonic or ego-dystonic? What about obsessive compulsive personality disorder?	OCD is ego-dystonic. OCPD is egosyntonic.
☐ Describe the result of a Weber hearing test in a patient with conductive hearing loss.	Patient will report the sound louder in the affected ear.
☐ What is the treatment for myxedema?	Levothyroxine and slow warming
☐ What is the treatment for a bad brown recluse spider bite?	Debridement, the venom causes tissue necrosis.
☐ Define paraphimosis	Foreskin is retracted and cannot be reduced.
☐ Are the lungs noisy or quiet in COPD?	Quiet
☐ Name three medications used to break a seizure?	Diazepam, lorazepam, phenytoin or fosphenytoin
☐ At how many weeks of pregnancy can an amniocentesis be done?	15-20 weeks
☐ A painless, clean base chancre should make you think of what diagnosis?	Primary syphilis

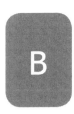

A 60 year old male presents to the ER with severe dizziness and back pain. His blood pressure is dropping, and you can feel an abdominal pulsatile mass on physical exam. What is the most likely diagnosis?	Ruptured aortic aneurysm
Are ulcers from arterial insufficiency painful or painless?	Painful
What is the most common location of colorectal cancer?	Cecum about 38%
You notice drusen deposits on fundal exam. What diagnosis should you be thinking of?	Macular degeneration
A description of a young girl with a web neck or wide shield chest should make you think of what diagnosis?	Turner's syndrome
Define stage 1 hypertension according to JNC 7.	Systolic pressure of 140-159 and diastolic of 90-99
A patient has had GERD for years. Over the past year, he has noticed an increase in difficulty swallowing his food. This should make you think of what diagnosis?	Esophageal strictures
An elderly patient presents with dyspnea, angina and syncope on exertion. The EKG is normal. What is the most likely diagnosis?	Aortic stenosis
A Patient presents with progressive neck and proximal muscle weakness. On physical exam, you see a reddish purple maculopapular rash. Her lab work shows an anti-Jo-1 antibodies. What is the most likely diagnosis?	Polymyositis
Name three serious reactoins a patient may have with the use of vancomycin?	Nephrotoxicity, ototoxicity and Stevens-Johnson syndrome

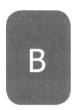

☐	Which of the four rotator cuff muscles is most commonly injured?	Supraspinatus
☐	What uric acid level helps to confirm a diagnosis of gout?	>7.5
☐	At what age should an infant begin cooing?	2 months
☐	Vasculitis with a hepatitis B history should make you think of what diagnosis?	Polyarteritis nodosa
☐	What lab test is the gold standard for chlamydia?	Nucleic acid amplification test
☐	What are the first three steps of managing pancreatitis?	NPO, pain control, fluids
☐	Depigmented patches of skin should make you think of what diagnosis?	Vitiligo
☐	A patient presents with a lateralized throbbing headache. He is also complaining of nausea, vomiting and photophobia. What type of headache is most likely?	Migraine
☐	A low retic count and a normal serum ferritin should make you think of what diagnosis?	Anemia of chronic disease
☐	Where on your patient should you listen for the murmur associated with an atrial septal defect?	At the left second or third interspace.
☐	In order to diagnose rheumatic fever what one thing must you have?	Evidence of a strep infection either positive titer or positive culture. In addition to that you need 2 major criteria or 1 major and 2 minor criteria.

On an EKG, you notice a patient has a gradually lengthening PR interval and then a missed QRS complex. The pattern repeats again. What type of AV block is this?	*Mobitz I or Wenckebach*
List three positive symptoms of schizophrenia.	*Hallucinations, delusions, movement disorders*
Calf pain should always make you think of what diagnosis?	*DVT*
A 15 year old boy presents complaining of night pain in the pelvis. Since you have no idea what to do, you order an x-ray. The report comes back with a description of a mass with an "onion skin appearance." What is the most likely diagnosis?	*Ewing sarcoma*
An EEG showing focal rhythmic discharges at the onset of the seizure should make you think of what diagnosis?	*Simple partial seizure*
Carpal tunnel affects what nerve and what parts of the hand?	*Median nerve. Thumb, pointer and ring fingers. Thenar wasting is sign of advanced disease.*
A patient is having seizures along with a mouse-like odor from the urine. What diagnosis should you be thinking of?	*Phenylketonuria*
Define phimosis.	*Foreskin can not be retracted.*
How do you treat vaginal candida?	*Fluconazole po 1 dose or azole cream x 1 week*
A leukemia patient has a CT of the liver which shows punched out lesions. What diagnosis should you be thinking of?	*Hepatosplenic candida*

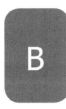

☐	What is Reynold's pentad and why does it matter?	Charcot's triad + hypotension + altered mental status. It indicates high risk of sepsis.
☐	Vaginal infection with motile flagellated protozoa should make you think of what diagnosis?	Trichomonas vaginitis
☐	If you are looking for lesions associated with multiple sclerosis and you order an MRI do you order with gadolinium or without?	With gadolinium
☐	How does nicotinic acid work to affect the lipid profile?	It inhibits secretion of VLDL
☐	After 7 days of sinusitis what antibiotic would you start?	Amoxicillin or Bactrim
☐	What organism is most commonly responsible for community acquired pneumonia?	Strep pneumoniae
☐	Bat wing vessels or Kerley B lines on a CXR should make you think of what diagnosis?	CHF
☐	Painless bright red blood per rectum should make you think of what diagnosis?	Hemorrhoids
☐	What is Schilling's test used for?	Test for the cause of a B12 deficiency.
☐	German measles is also known as what disease?	Rubella
☐	What is the treatment for most Mallory-Weiss tears?	Watchful waiting, these will typically resolve within 48 hours.
☐	A string sign on barium swallow should make you think of what diagnosis?	Pyloric stenosis
☐	Which four human papillomaviruses are linked to cervical cancer?	HPV 16, 18, 31 and 33
☐	Propranolol belongs to what class of medication?	Beta blockers

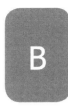

☐ How do you treat a patient with respiratory syncytial virus?	*Albuterol, steroids and fluids*
☐ A 22 year old male patient presents with what is clearly a septic knee. You also notice lesions on his hands and feet. What is the most likely pathogen?	*Neisseria gonorrhoeae*
☐ Define menorrhagia.	*Heavy prolonged menstrual flow*
☐ Which finding requires immediate attention: left bundle branch block or right bundle branch block?	*New left bundle branch block is a STEMI equivalent. Right bundle branch block is usually not a problem.*
☐ What is the most common type of testicular cancer?	*Non-seminoma*
☐ What is the most common vessel blocked with intestinal ischemia?	*Superior mesenteric artery*
☐ On auscultation, you hear a harsh, blowing, pansystolic murmur at the apex. What is the most likely diagnosis?	*Mitral regurgitation*
☐ What disease does Rickettsia rickettsii cause?	*Rocky Mountain spotted fever*
☐ Projectile vomiting should make you think of what diagnosis?	*Pyloric stenosis*
☐ What treatment should be started for asymptomatic diverticulosis?	*None*
☐ 46 year old male comes into ER limping a little on the right side. He states that it felt as though he was kicked in the back of the leg during a soccer game, but clearly no one was behind him. What is the most likely diagnosis?	*Achilles tendon rupture*
☐ Scleroderma limited version has five main characteristics for which the CREST acronym is often used. What are those five things?	*Calcinosis, Raynaud's, esophageal dysmotility, Sclerodactyly, Telangiectasia*

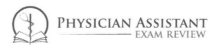

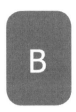

☐ What two human papillomaviruses are most responsible for condyloma acuminata?	HPV 6 and 11
☐ A patient complains of having suddenly developed stage fright. It is very important to his career that he be able to speak in front of groups. What medication might you treat him with?	Beta blocker - propranolol
☐ Lead I has a QRS that is up and the AVF lead has a QRS complex that is down. Does this represent normal axis, left axis deviation or right axis deviation?	Left axis deviation
☐ Any reference to dark field microscopy should make you think of what organism?	Treponema pallidum
☐ A patient presents drooling, with stridor and in tripod position. What is the diagnosis, and how do you treat it?	You treat epiglottitis with a second or third generation cephalosporin like cefuroxime or ceftriaxone.
☐ Purple, pruritic, polygonal, papules on physical exam should make you think of what diagnosis?	Lichen planus
☐ How long after a radiant energy burn do symptoms typically show?	6-12 hours
☐ A patient of yours always craves attention, often using sex as a tool to gain it. She often acts like a child when she does not get her way? What diagnosis should you be thinking of?	Histrionic personality disorder
☐ What is the most specific test for acute cholecystitis?	HIDA
☐ How long does menstruation need to be absent before secondary amenorrhea can be diagnosed?	If cycles have been previously normal: 3 months. If cycles have been previously irregular: 6 months.
☐ What area of the prostate is affected by BPH?	The transitional zone

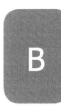

The term Philadelphia chromosome should make you think of what diagnosis?	Chronic myeloid leukemia
What dermatologic finding is associated with insulin insensitivity?	Acanthosis nigricans
What is the treatment for pertussis?	Erythromycin x 7 days
What is the treatment for a patient with a Mobitz II AV block?	Pacemaker
Diarrhea with blood and mucus should make you think of what diagnosis?	Shigella
A patient presents with pain in one eye. The cornea is hazy and the pupils are fixed. What is the most likely diagnosis?	Glaucoma
What is pertussis more commonly referred to as?	Whooping cough
What are two things that an anal fissure off midline might suggest?	Crohn's, syphilis, HIV, neoplasm
Does niacin increase or decrease HDL?	Increase
What are the 5 points of Ranson's criteria on admission?	older than 55, WBC>16, glucose>200, LDH>350, AST>250
Nodular opacities in the upper lung fields should make you think of what diagnosis?	Silicosis
Pitting nails are associated with what dermatologic disorder?	Psoriasis
Where do most aortic dissections occur?	The ascending or descending thoracic aorta
Tapioca blisters should make you think of what diagnosis?	Dyshidrosis - these are usually on the hands and feet.

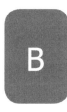

☐ Describe how to perform the obturator sign.	*The patient is supine and attempts to flex and internally rotate right hip.*
☐ What characteristic of pelvic inflammatory disease will help to differentiate it in a question stem from ectopic pregnancy, appendicitis, ovarian torsion and ovarian cyst?	*It will be bilateral pain. Most other common abdominal complaints have unilateral pain.*
☐ Since a genetic cause is the number one reason for primary amenorrhea what is one very important test?	*Karyotype*
☐ Which are painful and found on the fingers and toes, Osler nodes or Janeway lesions?	*Osler nodes*
☐ Atypical or walking pneumonia is caused by what pathogen?	*Mycoplasma*
☐ What is the most common congenital heart disease?	*Ventricular septal defect*
☐ What medicaton classes are prescribed in order to help prevent chronic renal failure in diabetic patients?	*ACEIs or ARBs*
☐ An EKG shows two premature ventricular contractions. These two QRS waves look very different. What is the term for this?	*Multifocal premature ventricular contractions*
☐ What are the three major criteria for endocarditis?	*2 positive blood cultures, a positive transesophageal echocardiography, new murmur*
☐ Exophthalmos should make you think of what diagnosis?	*Hyperthyroidism*
☐ You see a short PR interval and a delta wave on EKG. What is the most likely diagnosis?	*Wolff-Parkinson-White syndrome*

B

If you hear a midsystolic click you should immediately be thinking about what diagnosis?	Mitral valve prolapse
In Cushing's disease is ACTH elevated or decreased?	Elevated
Weakness and numbness in the left hand might be a blockage in which carotid artery?	Right
What is included in Whipple's triad of hypoglycemia?	History of previous hypoglycemia, serum glucose of <40, immediate recovery upon administration of glucose
Which problem is an emergency phimosis or paraphimosis?	Paraphimosis
List three congenital heart diseases.	Atrial septal defect (ASD), ventricular septal defect (VSD), coarctation of the aorta, patent ductus arteriosus (PDA), tetralogy of Fallot
What is the first line medical treatment for a pheochromocytoma?	Alpha blockers
What is the most common cause of postpartum hemorrhage?	Uterine atony
What medication can be used to control bleeding due to uterine atony?	Oxytocin (Pitocin)
A 16 year old has just moved schools. He is quiet, moody and not like himself at all. Within six months he seems to have completely changed back to his previous personality. What diagnosis should you be thinking of?	Adjustment disorder
What is the most common sexually transmitted bacteria?	Chlamydia

B

☐	What is the medical term for lazy eye?	*Amblyopia*
☐	Acute sinusitis is most commonly caused by which two pathogens?	*Strep pneumoniae and haemophilus influenzae*
☐	Rhinophyma should make you think of what diagnosis?	*Acne rosacea*
☐	A Westermark sign on CXR should make you think of what diagnosis?	*Pulmonary embolism*
☐	Positive antithyroid peroxidase and antithyroglobulin antibodies should make you think of what diagnosis ?	*Hashimoto's*
☐	What are two tocolytic medications you should be aware of?	*Magnesium sulfate and calcium channel blockers*
☐	Would anemia of chronic disease most likely be macrocytic, normocytic or microcytic?	*Normocytic*
☐	How do you definitively diagnose rabies?	*Pathology of the brain of the animal that performed the bite using fluorescent antibody stain.*
☐	List four symptoms of serotonin syndrome.	*Hyperthermia!, seizure, mental status change, tremor*
☐	What should a primary care provider do for presumed central retinal artery occlusion?	*Ophthalmic emergency! Refer and intermittent pressure and release of the eye.*
☐	What is the treatment for subconjunctival hemorrhage?	*Reassurance*
☐	What are three possible treatments for peritonsillar abscess?	*Needle aspiration, I&D and tonsillectomy*

B

What does an Anti-HBc (hep B core antibody) indicate?	Previous or ongoing hepatitis B infection
An EKG shows a regular rate of 50 beats per minute. The QRS is narrow and there is no visible P wave. What is the most likely diagnosis?	Junctional rythm
A patient presents to the ER with tearing chest pain radiating to his back. What is the most likely diagnosis?	Aortic dissection
Describe the psoas sign.	The patient is supine and attempts to raise the right leg against resistance.
Under normal conditions at what hemoglobin level would you begin to consider a transfusion?	8
What is the most common cause of an atrial septal defect?	Patent foramen ovale
White curd like vaginal discharge should make you think of what diagnosis?	Vaginal candida infection
The scotch tape test is used to diagnose what disease?	Pinworm
A patient is brought in following a seizure in which she did not lose consciousness. What diagnosis should you be thinking of?	Simple partial seizure
What is the most common cause of hypopituitarism?	Tumor
What are the two most common causes of pancreatitis?	Cholelithiasis and ETOH
A positive straight leg test indicates what diagnosis?	Herniated disc

B

☐	What is the main function of parathyroid hormone?	*Increase serum Ca*
☐	A bamboo spine indicates what diagnosis?	*Ankylosing spondylitis*
☐	A patient presents following a seizure. Just before the siezure she remembers seeing flashing lights all around her. What diagnosis should be at the top of your differential?	*Complex partial*
☐	Define paradoxical pulse.	*There is a large difference in pulse pressure between inhalation and exhalation.*
☐	Honeycombing and tram tracks on the CXR should make you think of what diagnosis?	*Bronchiectasis and idopathic pulmonary fibrosis*
☐	How is celiac disease most commonly diagnosed?	*Endoscopic biopsy*
☐	Which heart valve is most associated with rheumatic fever?	*Mitral*
☐	A patient presents to the ER after taking a baseball bat to the knee. He is unable to actively extend his knee. What is the most likely diagnosis?	*Patella fracture*
☐	What is the first thing you should be thinking of if a pediatric patient comes in with blood in the anterior chamber of the eye (hyphema).	*Child abuse until proven otherwise*
☐	What is the treatment for a tetanus infections?	*Penicillin, immune globulin and supportive care (especially respiratory support)*
☐	What type of hearing loss would be caused by cerumen impaction?	*Conductive*
☐	What are four steps in treating diphtheria?	*Antitoxin, penicillin, remove membrane, report the case to the CDC*

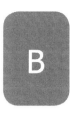

List three possible causes of prerenal renal failure.	CHF, severe dehydration, hemorrhage
List four risk factors for breast cancer?	BRCA1 or BRCA2 positive, unopposed estrogen, nulliparity, early menarche, late menopause
What are the two main complications of cirrhosis?	Portal HTN & liver insufficiency
Which viral exanthem often has conjunctivitis as one of it's symptoms?	Measles/Rubeola
A spiral fracture should make you think of what issue?	Abuse, either child or elder
Unilateral purulent rhinitis should make you think of what diagnosis?	Foreign body
How do you treat a sickle cell crisis?	Fluids, oxygen, pain medication, transfusion may be necessary
Tenderness over the anatomical snuffbox is indicative of what fracture?	Scaphoid
What is the only cyanotic congenital heart disease on the NCCPA blueprint?	Tetralogy of Fallot
Will the RBC's be large, small or normal size in a B12 deficient anemia?	Macrocytes
A patient describes his vision loss as curtain coming down and then going back up. What might the diagnosis be?	Amaurosis fugax
What is the treatment for epiglottitis?	2nd or 3rd generation cephalosporins (ceftriaxone), macrolides may also be used (clindamycin)

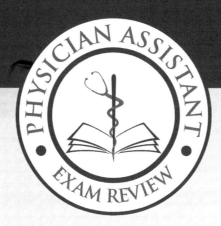

Your confidence should be sky high at this point. If you get the key terms in this book, then you have an excellent foundation for the exam. Make sure you get eight hours of sleep the night before, and please let me know how you do.

You can reach out to me at:

✉ bwallace@physicianassistantexamreview.com

or leave your story along with hundreds of others at:

🖱 www.physicianassistantexamreview.com/yourstory

There is tons of free additional review material at:

🖱 **www.physicianassistantexamreview.com**

including podcasts covering every topic on the NCCPA blueprint, notes, study tips and even more questions.

Good luck.